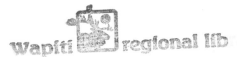

ACTION PLAN FOR

HIGH BLOOD PRESSURE

ACTION PLAN FOR
HIGH BLOOD PRESSURE

JON G. DIVINE, MD

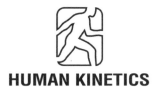

HUMAN KINETICS

Library of Congress Cataloging-in-Publication Data

Divine, Jon G.
  Action plan for high blood pressure / Jon G. Divine
       p. cm.
  Includes bibliographical references and index.
  ISBN 0-7360-5140-6 (soft cover)
  1.   Hypercholesteremia--Popular works. 2.   Blood cholesterol--Popular works.
I. Title.
  RC632.H83D58 2005
  616.3'997--dc22

                                                          2005017320

ISBN: 0-7360-5140-6

Acquisitions Editor: Martin Barnard; **Developmental Editor:** Leigh Keylock; **Copyeditor:** Jacqueline Eaton Blakley; **Proofreader:** Jim Burns; **Indexer:** Betty Frizzéll; **Permission Manager:** Carly Breeding; **Graphic Designer:** Fred Starbird; **Graphic Artist:** Tara Welsch; **Photo Manager:** Dan Wendt; **Cover Designer:** Jack W. Davis; **Photographer (interior):** Dan Wendt, unless otherwise noted; **Art Manager:** Kareema McLendon-Foster; **Printer:** United Graphics

ACSM Publication Committee Chair: Jeffrey L. Roitman, EdD, FACSM; **ACSM Communications and Public Information Committee Chair:** Harold W. Kohl, PhD, FACSM; **ACSM Group Publisher:** D. Mark Robertson; **ACSM Editorial Manager:** Lori A. Tish

We thank Body Tech in St. Joseph, Illinois, for assistance in providing the location for the photo shoot for this book.

Human Kinetics books are available at special discounts for bulk purchase. Special editions or book excerpts can also be created to specification. For details, contact the Special Sales Manager at Human Kinetics.

Printed in the United States of America   10   9   8   7   6   5   4   3   2   1

Human Kinetics
Web site: www.HumanKinetics.com

United States: Human Kinetics
P.O. Box 5076
Champaign, IL 61825-5076
800-747-4457
e-mail: humank@hkusa.com

Canada: Human Kinetics
475 Devonshire Road Unit 100
Windsor, ON N8Y 2L5
800-465-7301 (in Canada only)
e-mail: orders@hkcanada.com

Europe: Human Kinetics
107 Bradford Road
Stanningley
Leeds LS28 6AT, United Kingdom
+44 (0) 113 255 5665
e-mail: hk@hkeurope.com

Australia: Human Kinetics
57A Price Avenue
Lower Mitcham, South Australia 5062
08 8277 1555
e-mail: liaw@hkaustralia.com

New Zealand: Human Kinetics
Division of Sports Distributors NZ Ltd.
P.O. Box 300 226 Albany
North Shore City
Auckland
0064 9 448 1207
e-mail: info@humankinetics.co.nz

To Evan, Ryan, and Leigh Ann—three pats.

CONTENTS

ACKNOWLEDGMENTS

This book was a little scary, yet fun, to put together. After agreeing to write this book, in order to be closer to my family in the Midwest and to take on a new career challenge, I accepted a position in Cincinnati, and moved there from Houston. Once the dust settled and the last few boxes were unpacked, I was able to resume writing. Through the period of personal transition, the staff at Human Kinetics was patient, encouraging, and overall great to work with. Special thanks go to Leigh Keylock, Developmental Editor, for her patience, encouragement, and excellent editorial work. Leigh's encouraging e-mails and reminders were the one constant in the whole process. Thanks for everything, Leigh. Additional thanks go to Acquisitions Editor Martin Barnard, and to the entire production staff at Human Kinetics for their work on this project. Additional thanks to my "coauthor," the American College of Sports Medicine—specifically, D. Mark Robertson and Lori Tish. Most of all, thanks go to my good friend Bill Kohl, who has been instrumental in all of my administrative work with ACSM, and who had a guiding hand (and editing pen) in establishing my involvement with this project.

Jessie Owens once said, "Nobody ever gains the pinnacle of success unless he has somebody helping him along the way. You don't do it alone." I have been very lucky in my life to have had the guiding hand of many individuals, coaches, and mentors, "helping me along the way." Those include teachers and coaches—Chuck Deyo, Steve Kull, Bruce Smith, Al Simpson, and Guido Ricevuto—who taught me the value of hard work at an influential age and who left me with the lasting memory that everything worthwhile in life is worth working hard for—and if it wasn't, then everyone would have it and it wouldn't be worth anything. We shared many times of hard work that were fun at the same time—even if the short-term pay-off was not perfect, the life lesson learned was the most important.

It's always good to acknowledge and thank the people whom you work with (and for) everyday. Special thanks to Drs. Tom Boat, Jeff Robbins, and Tim Hewett, who provided me with an opportunity in 2003 to help create a great environment to practice medicine at Cincinnati Children's Hospital in our new Sports Medicine Biodynamics Center. Also to the truly great group of dedicated people I see every day—thank you to all, especially Tiffany Evans and RN-extraordinaire Jo Ford for their daily assistance.

Thanks should also go to John Lombardo who taught me that knowing is important but being able to convey knowledge, especially to patients or colleagues, is *very important.* John is a great doctor, one of the "founding fathers" of primary care sports medicine, but he is an even better teacher, especially in educating patients and their loved ones. I owe a lot to John for what he taught me.

My parents, R.J. and Diana Divine, have provided me with a lifetime of simple lessons and have always done it with their unconditional love and support. I could never thank them enough.

Finally, thanks to all of my past and present patients (especially those who allowed me to use their stories in this book). You all have taught me more from the privilege of providing your care than any textbook.

INTRODUCTION

Picture this. Near the end of an office visit to decide how to manage a newly diagnosed illness, your doctor prescribes medication.

"You should take this medicine. It's good for you," your physician advises.

"How much should I take?" you ask.

"Well, about as much as you feel like that day."

"And how often should I take it?"

"Frequently. Try to take it every day, if you can."

Doesn't sound like very effective advice, does it?

Because physicians are generally not trained very well in exercise science, this can be a common discussion script when they advise patients about regular exercise. For years, we have known the positive influence of exercise and regular physical activity on blood pressure and the illness of hypertension. We know which types of exercises abnormally raise blood pressure acutely and which types and amounts of exercise chronically lower blood pressure. The journal *The Physician and Sportsmedicine* has been telling us for years that "exercise is medicine."

We can even go so far as to say that there is a dose-related influence of exercise on most illnesses. Unfortunately, the emphasis in recent years has been to determine the minimum amount of activity necessary to receive any benefit from exercise, rather than how to receive the maximum benefit from exercise on a given condition or illness. This is the underlying emphasis of this book: how to achieve the maximum benefit in blood pressure control from exercise. Consider this book your owner's manual for actively reducing your blood pressure. Each chapter ends with a checklist of points you will take with you from the chapter, which will help you develop your "action plan."

In the first chapter we try to define in simple terms what it means to have high blood pressure, or hypertension. These two terms are used interchangeably throughout this book. In order to make a medical diagnosis of hypertension, your doctor will follow a simple but important series of procedures to determine your resting blood pressure. If you have three consecutive elevated blood pressure readings, your doctor will then determine the best course of management to reduce your resting pressure. Certainly exercise will be an important component in your plan. Chapter 2 explains how regular exercise influences your blood pressure and introduces the FITT concept of exercise as medication.

During your initial visits to the doctor's office, you will be asked to do a few other tests—specifically, blood tests looking for other conditions such as elevated cholesterol or elevated blood sugar, which occur together in many people with high blood pressure. Because your heart health determines your pressure, and vice versa, it will also be essential to determine whether there are any current problems or risks of future problems with your pump function. Chapter 3 reviews what to expect during your initial visits to the doctor's office and explains what tests are done. Of equal importance, you will learn how to do several self-assessments of your current fitness level. Descriptions of how to perform several self-assessments of aerobic capacity, flexibility, and strength are included. This information will be the basis for how to individualize your personal fitness program and is perhaps some of the most important information in the book.

Chapter 4 goes into further detail about how aerobic fitness improves blood pressure, in addition to providing practical information about participation in team and individual sports, preventing injury, choosing exercise apparel, and factors influencing what time of day to exercise. Sample programs for walking, running, cycling, and swimming are detailed. Chapters 5 and 6 discuss the importance of regular strength and flexibility training. Advice on specific strength and flexibility training techniques and sample programs are included.

Again, the goal of this book is to provide you with self-empowering information that will allow you to take an active role in controlling your blood pressure. The first step in the medical management of hypertension is for you and your doctor to make an active plan to make the necessary lifestyle modifications that can help reduce your elevated blood pressure. The focus of this text is on how to maximize the use of exercise in your modification plan. Chapter 7 brings together the various lifestyle modifications that can reduce blood pressure, shows you how your doctor decides what is best for you, and reviews important diet information. The DASH diet, a diet proven to help reduce blood pressure, is highlighted. The pros and cons of other in-vogue diets are also discussed.

By not smoking, losing weight, reducing sodium, following a heart-smart diet, reducing alcohol consumption, and of course increasing your amount of daily physical activity, you can reduce your blood pressure anywhere from 5 to 20 mmHg! If you have been newly diagnosed with prehypertension (at risk of later hypertension) or with mildly elevated (stage 1 or 2) pressure, your doctor will strongly encourage you to make these lifestyle modifications before beginning medication therapy. The amount of time will be based on how high your pressure is.

If you have additional health problems, such as heart disease, diabetes, or kidney disease, or if your pressure is considerably elevated, your doctor has probably already prescribed medication to begin to reduce your blood pressure. Chapter 7 also covers the influence of blood pressure medications on exercise. Current recommendations regarding which medications are best for managing blood pressure have been well researched. However, very few studies have included subjects who were active exercisers. That is why you should take a few moments to read about which class of medications may have been prescribed for you and to learn how your medication could affect your ability to exercise. The information may surprise you and could stimulate conversation during your next visit with your physician.

Because hypertension is a chronic disease, it will require your attention for the remainder of your life. Although for many this sounds intimidating and depressing, it can be viewed as another of life's challenges to be conquered. You will more than likely make significant strides toward improving your blood pressure by following the advice on exercise and activity in this book. Once you have finished the book, don't let your enthusiasm die. Chapter 8 has specific tips to help you not only stay with your program, but improve as well.

This is one of those first steps in a thousand-mile journey. Don't fret, don't panic, and don't look at the journey as long—this will add to your pressure! Remember, when you follow this advice, you are seizing a health situation presumably out of your control and actually taking control. Enjoy the ride.

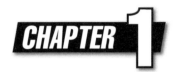
WINNING THE BLOOD PRESSURE BATTLE

According to the Seventh Report of the Joint National Committee on Prevention, Detection, Evaluation, and Treatment of High Blood Pressure, 58 million Americans (29 percent of the population) have high blood pressure, or *hypertension* (Chobanian et al. 2003). This represents a 30 percent increase over the previous decade. According to the American Heart Association (2005), approximately 4 out of 10 African-Americans have high blood pressure, compared with about 3 out of 10 Mexican-Americans and Caucasians.

Hypertension is the third most common reason people visit their family physician's office and the number-one abnormal finding on annual health exams across all age ranges. The number of Americans with high blood pressure is steadily increasing—particularly in the adolescent population, which is also seeing a rapid rise in obesity. In fact, obesity and high blood pressure combine to create one of the most common tandems of illness in the U.S. Of adolescents who have a blood pressure of 142/90 on a preparticipation sports exam, 80 percent will go on to have adult hypertension. Based on these results, we can expect the number of people with hypertension in America to rise dramatically in the next 20 to 30 years.

It's no surprise that the number of Americans who are obese or overweight correlates with the number of Americans who do not get enough exercise. So it certainly makes sense that exercise is good for people with hypertension who are overweight—in fact, every 10 pounds lost generates a 10 percent reduction in blood pressure. But even more exciting is that the beneficial effects of regular exercise lower chronically high blood pressure *independent of weight loss*. With regular exercise training, resting (as opposed to exercising) systolic pressure goes down and stays down, as long as you stay active. And people who exercise regularly manage stress better, have a better outlook on life, sleep better, describe the feeling of having more energy, and generally feel better.

Systolic and Diastolic Pressures

For years, high blood pressure has been referred to as the "silent killer" because it often develops with few or no symptoms. Usually, other than having a family history of high blood pressure, a person who has this condition has no indication of its existence, although hypertension can lead to several additional health problems that do have symptoms. We do know the risk factors, however, that increase the likelihood of hypertension, and these are the following:

- Family history of high blood pressure
- Diabetes or kidney disease
- African-American heritage
- Male
- Age (35 years and older)
- Smoking
- Obesity
- Use of oral birth control medication
- Excessive alcohol consumption (more than two drinks per day)
- Sedentary lifestyle

One of the few indications that blood pressure may be going up—weight gain—should prompt you not only to check blood pressure at least annually, but to do so as a part of a regular physical exam by your personal physician.

Say your blood pressure is 140/90. The top number, 140, is the *systolic* pressure. This is the pressure in the arteries leading from the heart as the heart is pumping. The bottom number, 90, is the *diastolic* pressure, or the pressure in the arteries when the heart is resting for the few microseconds between beats.

Both pressures are important. For a long time it was believed that rising systolic pressure was a normal part of aging. Some may remember hearing that a normal systolic pressure was 120 plus your age! We now know that this is false and that blood pressure should not go up as a result of the natural, healthy aging process. Changes in systolic blood pressure with aging are the result of stiffening of the arteries, which occurs gradually as the arteries protect themselves against—you guessed it—steadily rising blood pressure.

In the past 20 years, diastolic pressure has received more attention in doctors' offices because it was thought to be related to a higher incidence of complications due to high blood pressure, such as heart disease, stroke, and kidney disease. More recent studies of large populations indicate that those with systolic pressures greater than 140 are as much at risk of these same complications as those with chronically elevated diastolic pressures above 90. Therefore, it is important to identify and control elevations in both pressures.

Diastolic pressure normally goes down during exercise. As with systolic pressure, resting diastolic blood pressure goes down because of regular exercise and activity. It can go up during exercise; when it does, it is one of the first signs that hypertension is (or will be) present. This certainly does not mean you should stop exercising; on the contrary, it means you should be exercising more regularly.

Measurement and Interpretation of Blood Pressure

Several factors affect the accuracy of blood pressure measurement, including who is measuring—pressure readings in doctors' offices are notoriously elevated in people with "white coat hypertension," probably because those people don't like being in a doctor's office! The blood pressure cuff size also can influence the measured pressure by as much as 10 percent. A blood pressure cuff should fit snugly but should not feel too tight around the upper arm. For accurate measurement of blood pressure, larger people require larger cuff sizes. The time of day can also influence pressure. Generally, pressures are higher during the morning hours, then decrease somewhat throughout the day, then increase slightly later in the afternoon and evening.

Given this variability, how can you be sure that your elevated blood pressure reading is indeed hypertension? By having your pressure measured at rest, on three separate occasions, spread apart by at least a day, you can be sure that consistently elevated blood pressure is a real finding and does indicate hypertension.

One technique gaining popularity is 24-hour, or *ambulatory,* monitoring of blood pressure. With this technique, the individual wears a less bulky but appropriately sized blood pressure cuff that monitors changes in blood pressure during a 24-hour period. This virtually eliminates so-called white coat hypertension, which can be the cause of up to 20 percent of abnormally elevated readings. In addition, ambulatory monitoring can detect failure of blood pressure to decrease 10 to 20 percent during sleep, which is associated with a greater risk of organ damage, including heart disease. With these data in hand, your physician can review with you the highs and lows of the day that influence your blood pressure. It can be very insightful to see that a tense conversation with your brother-in-law or your morning commute in heavy traffic really did raise your pressure.

Table 1.1 can help you determine the severity of your pressure readings. Again, risk of complications due to high blood pressure, such as heart attacks, stroke, and kidney damage, go up as your resting pressure goes up. How your doctor will advise you on managing your blood pressure will be discussed in later chapters; ideally, a doctor should encourage you not only to take a more active role in controlling your blood pressure but also to *be more active* to control your blood pressure.

Table 1.1   Classification of Hypertension in Adults

Class	Systolic blood pressure	Diastolic blood pressure
Optimal	<120	<80
Normal	<130	<85
Prehypertensive	130–139	85–89
Hypertension		
Stage 1	140–159	90–99
Stage 2	160–179	100–109
Stage 3	>180	>110

Adapted from A.V. Chobanian, G.L. Bakris, H.R. Black, et al. 2003. "The seventh report of the Joint National Committee on Prevention, Detection, Evaluation, and Treatment of High Blood Pressure: the JNC 7 report." *Journal of the American Medical Association* 289: 2560-2572.

Hypertension in Children and Adolescents

The definition of young gets older every day, but for our purposes let's define *young* as under 42 years old. Blood pressure in children should be lower than blood pressure in late adolescents and adults. The ranges of severity of hypertension for children 6 to 18 years of age are listed in table 1.2; note that a normal adult blood pressure of 120/80 would be considered high for a 10-year-old. Unfortunately, we are witnessing an alarming trend of both obesity and elevated blood pressure in the youngest populations. Of the adolescents with pressures greater than 142/90 on annual physical exams, 80 percent will eventually develop chronic hypertension as adults. It's vital to try to identify and correct this problem as early in life as possible. Again, an annual checkup that includes appropriate measurement of blood pressure is essential for every child (especially for those who are overweight).

Table 1.2   Severity of Hypertension in Children and Adolescents

Age/severity	Systolic blood pressure	Diastolic blood pressure	Activity restrictions
6 to 9 years			
Mild	120–124	75–79	None
Moderate	125–129	80–84	None
Severe	130–139	85–89	Control needed before exercise
Very severe	>140	>90	Control needed before exercise
10 to 12 years			
Mild	125–129	80–84	None
Moderate	130–134	85–89	None
Severe	135–144	90–94	Control needed before exercise
Very severe	>145	>95	Control needed before exercise
13 to 15 years			
Mild	135–139	85–89	None
Moderate	140–149	90–94	None
Severe	150–159	95–99	Control needed before exercise
Very severe	>160	>100	Control needed before exercise
16 to 18 years			
Mild	140–149	90–94	None
Moderate	150–159	95–99	None
Severe	160–179	100–109	Control needed before exercise
Very severe	>180	>110	Control needed before exercise

Adapted from A.V. Chobanian, G.L. Bakris, H.R. Black, et al. 2003. "The seventh report of the Joint National Committee on Prevention, Detection, Evaluation, and Treatment of High Blood Pressure: the JNC 7 report." *Journal of the American Medical Association* 289: 2560-2572.

The incidence of syndrome X (obesity, hypertension, and insulin resistance) in those younger than 18 years is approaching 30 percent. Once thought to be a disease process seen only in adults, insulin resistance, along with obesity and high blood pressure, is on the rise in children and adolescents. Before 1990, this combination was rarely seen in the young.

Characteristics of young persons at highest risk include the following:

- African-American heritage
- Obesity
- Family history of diabetes or hypertension
- Personal or family history of kidney disease
- Previous spinal cord injury

Causes of Hypertension

Ninety-five percent of the time, we do not know the cause of hypertension. Several theories exist: hardening and lost compliance (stretchability) of the arteries; increased tone of the smooth muscle lining of the arteries; perhaps slowed kidney function resulting in fluid and sodium retention. Whatever the theory, the result is definite: the pressure in the arteries is chronically elevated and will lead to disastrous results if left unchecked.

What about the other 5 percent? These causes are referred to as *secondary* causes of hypertension. Although these causes are rare, the initial tests done on patients who are thought to have hypertension most often are done to rule out these secondary causes. Secondary causes also tend to result in very high pressure elevations: pressures of greater than 200/110 are not uncommon for those in this rare crowd. Secondary causes of hypertension are more common in younger people diagnosed with hypertension. The most common secondary causes include the following.

- **Sleep apnea.** Fifty percent of people with *sleep apnea* have hypertension. Most notice increased fatigue that concerns them enough to visit the doctor. Often, the first elevated pressure is measured at that point. Other common symptoms are falling asleep very easily during the day (even at stoplights while driving), loud snoring, and being overweight. Severe cases can result in right-sided heart failure and irregular heartbeats. If this sounds like you or a loved one, ask your doctor about having a sleep study. It could be a simple way to save your life.

- **Renal disease.** Usually the result of untreated high blood pressure and diabetes, *renal disease* occurs when vascular damage in the kidneys results in decreased ability to excrete salt and water, which in turn results in low plasma renin (a protein made by the kidneys that regulates body fluid) levels and retained fluid. The retained fluid increases the blood pressure, which causes a snowball effect of more damage to the kidneys.

- **Renal artery stenosis and renal vascular hypertension.** *Fibromuscular dysplasia* usually occurs in 25- to 50-year-olds and involves the formation of intravascular muscle in the distal renal artery that slows

Getting at the Root of the Pressure Problem

David was in his 40s and active, but he found his blood pressure and weight were rising. Despite being a coach and regular low-intensity exerciser, he could not lower his blood pressure, so he was put on medications. While he was on the medications, his blood pressure did not go down despite increases in dosage and the addition of a second medication, and his weight continued to go up. At a doctor's visit, David's wife commented strongly about his loud snoring keeping her awake, so the doctor suggested doing a sleep study. Through that study David discovered that he had severe sleep apnea, which caused him to stop breathing almost 40 times per hour while asleep, lowering his oxygen to dangerously low levels. Although this was going on nightly, he had been unaware of this potentially life-threatening problem. He began using a continuous positive air pressure (C-PAP) device while he slept. Almost immediately, he began to notice a difference in how he felt. He was less fatigued, woke up more rested, and his weight and blood pressure began to come down. Within six weeks he was taking only one blood pressure medication, at the lowest dose. With continued weight loss, he would probably be able to cease the medication altogether.

kidney function and worsens blood pressure. A similar process can occur in persons older than 50 who develop atherosclerosis (accumulation of plaque within the lining of the arteries) of renal arteries.

• **Adrenal hyperfunctioning.** Three different conditions occurring in the adrenal gland cause the adrenal gland to work "overtime," resulting in significantly higher blood pressure. Tumors of the adrenal gland—the tiny tissue "cap" on top of the kidneys—can result in elevated blood pressure. A *pheochromocytoma* secretes an excess amount of *catecholamines*, or stress hormones, resulting in not only very elevated blood pressure, but also high heart rate and sweating.

Cushing's disease results from an excess production of glucocorticoid steroids from the adrenal glands. This excess causes fluid retention, dramatic weight gain, fatigue, and skin changes.

Primary aldosteronism results in the retention of sodium and water because of excess aldosterone produced by the adrenal glands. This causes fluid retention, elevated blood pressure, and increased urinary excretion of potassium. Heartbeat irregularities and heart attacks can occur if the potassium levels drop too low.

• **Coarctation of the aorta.** This condition is a common secondary cause of elevated blood pressure in teenagers and is the result of a congenital narrowing of the aorta. Along with the irregular shape of the aorta, many smaller, or collateral, vessels form and can be seen on chest X-rays as "rib notching." Persons with this condition have elevated blood pressure when measured in the arms, but lower pressure when measured in the legs.

• **Hypothyroid.** Along with the classic changes associated with low thyroid levels such as weight gain, slowed metabolism, and fatigue, a decreased *cardiac output* (beat-by-beat volume of output from the heart) occurs, resulting in increased vascular tone. The smooth muscle lining of the blood vessels involuntarily contracts to maintain blood pressure at times when cardiac output decreases. This results in an elevation of resting blood pressure, usually the diastolic pressure.

• **Hyperthyroid.** Excessive thyroid hormone circulation results in an increase in cardiac output by increasing the heart rate and the force of contraction for each heart beat. This elevates systolic blood pressure, much like what occurs during exercise.

Dealing With Medication's Effects

Sue was a new member of the menopause club. Her doctor recommended hormone replacement therapy to reduce the hot flashes, fatigue, and sleeping problems she had been experiencing. Although she was active and not overweight, her blood pressure increased rapidly when she began taking the hormone replacement medications. Irritated from headaches, lack of sleep, and "more stress," she brought the bottle back to her doctor, wanting to stop taking the medicine that was making her feel so bad. The doctor realized a decimal point error had been made on the prescription, resulting in too much medication for Sue, and the appropriate dosage was then prescribed. Sue's symptoms improved but were still present even at an extremely low dose. She elected to come off the medications, and although she is still stressed sometimes, her blood pressure is perfect.

• **Decongestants and stimulants.** These drugs include over-the-counter cold and allergy medications, weight-loss medications, caffeine, and nicotine. During cold and flu season, many cases of elevated blood pressure are reported. This is simply because one of the key ingredients in over-the-counter decongestant medications can raise blood pressure. The same can be said for the now-banned diet medication ephedra. All act to increase both heart rate and the force of each heart contraction, which elevates blood pressure. The elevated pressure usually returns to normal levels once the medicine has metabolized and is out of the system.

• **NSAIDs and COX-2 inhibitors.** *Nonsteroidal anti-inflammatory drugs (NSAIDs)* can elevate the blood pressure of some individuals by affecting the fluid-excreting capacity of the kidneys. In susceptible individuals, pressure increases of 5 to 10 mmHg (millimeters of mercury, the standard unit of measure for blood pressure) have been observed. These pressure elevations have been reported to be irreversible in some. In more severe cases, this can result in irreversible kidney damage. There have been many cases of athletes who, partially dehydrated from exercise, took NSAIDs for relief of muscle pain and developed damage to the kidneys. Those with hypertension should use this group of drugs with caution especially at times of lower fluid levels as this is when the kidneys are most susceptible.*

- **Anabolic steroids.** In the quest to be bigger, perform better, and become stronger, athletes of all levels have discovered that taking anabolic steroids will help them meet these goals. Of course, this is not without a price—often, a high price. Taking anabolic steroids can result in larger skeletal muscles in addition to larger heart and blood vessel muscles. Larger heart muscles pump more blood per beat into blood vessels narrowed by contracted smooth muscles lining the vessels. Both these factors will raise blood pressure and can be irreversible. There are no reported ill effects on the kidneys, but the kidney is loaded with blood vessels that can be permanently damaged, resulting in elevated blood pressure for life. Anabolic steroids also increase cholesterol and triglyceride levels, further adding to the vascular pipe-clogging effects. Anyone with hypertension should not use anabolic steroids.

- **Anxiety and depression.** Americans in the workforce are constantly challenged to "do more with less." We have a greater sense of time urgency, have less free time and recreation, and live in a hostile culture. Although Americans work on our jobs more than citizens of any other country, we suffer from the highest amount of obesity and are plagued by diseases of inactivity. We compensate for stress either voluntarily or involuntarily by overeating. We drive farther to work. We have less time for recreation. And many of us do not manage well the stress we have created. Like many of the chronic conditions described earlier, this cultural environment may be irreversible. Thus, as our stress levels rise, our blood pressures rise as well. For many, the high blood pressure associated with acute stressful events remains elevated chronically. There are many theories as to why this occurs but no definite answers. Perhaps it is due to a higher frequency of adrenaline (catacholamine) release as a result of repetitive stressful events. It is known that individuals who live in densely populated areas, or who live next to areas of constant loud noise (highways, subways, or factories), have higher rates of hypertension.

*During the writing of this text, one form of COX-2 inhibitors, Celebrex, was still available to the public by prescription. Two (Bextra and Vioxx) had recently been pulled from the market because of the drugs' direct effects on blood pressure in some individuals and indirect effects on increased risk of heart attack death.

When Stress Rises, So Does Blood Pressure

Jean has a tough job: she is a spokesperson for a county health department. Part of her job is to stand in front of cameras and reassure the public when there are serious health issues in her community. She is also a single mom and grandparent, so her stress level does not improve when she leaves the office. Jean's blood pressure is extremely sensitive to her stress, but also comes down when she can relax. On two occasions, her pressures were very high in her doctor's office, so she was placed on medication to not only lower her pressure but also help her to manage stress better. Because the medication blocks her natural reactions to compensate for congenital anemia, Jean became chronically tired while taking the medications. Her doctor did not really understand what was going on until they agreed to do ambulatory monitoring. Despite having normal pressures in the doctor's office, her pressures became very low at various nonstressful times throughout the day. When she came off the medications, the pressures came up but she was less fatigued, so much so that she was able to step up her exercise routine and stabilize her pressures at a lower level. The stresses were still there, but mentally and physically she was better able to handle them when she was exercising regularly.

Conditions Resulting From Vascular Injury

Conditions resulting from vascular injury (end-organ damage) are those conditions commonly associated with hypertension. These include heart disease, stroke, retinopathy, and kidney disease and failure.

• **Heart disease.** Heart disease is the number-one cause of death in Americans. Hypertension, along with cigarette smoking, high cholesterol, and a sedentary lifestyle, are the lifestyle risk factors that have the greatest impact on the development of heart disease. In fact, every 20/10 mmHg increase in resting blood pressure above 115/75 doubles the risk of developing heart disease.

• **Stroke.** Anyone who has survived a stroke, or known someone who has, can certainly understand the potentially devastating effect on health and lifestyle caused by what can be a preventable event. It is estimated that up to one third of individuals with high blood pressure are not aware they have high blood pressure. This is probably because elevated pressures are usually asymptomatic—until it is too late, as is the case in strokes, or damage to areas of the brain caused by prolonged elevated blood pressure, which results in damage to the blood vessels supplying the brain. In these cases, no symptoms are usually present before the stroke or damage has been done. In addition, the blood pressure of up to one fourth of those on medication for high blood pressure is inadequately controlled by the prescribed medication. In both cases, it is crucial to have blood pressure checked regularly, to take medications as prescribed, and to follow up with your health care provider often.

• **Retinopathy.** Just as hypertension can damage vessels supplying the brain, it can also damage vessels to the retina, resulting in vision changes or blindness. Often, the damage can go unnoticed until it becomes irreversible.

• **Kidney disease and failure.** Elevated blood pressure is the leading cause of permanent kidney failure and the need for kidney transplants. Normal kidney function is intimately associated with normal blood pressure regulation. Perhaps no other organ in the body has so much control over an essential body function that can ultimately result in the destruction of itself and the body as a whole. The kidneys are loaded with blood vessels with internal mechanisms that recognize pressure fluctuations and adjust. In order to compensate for the acute pressure changes, these mechanisms can result in permanent changes in the vessels and organ as a whole.

How to Turn It Around

Once a diagnosis is established, you can work toward treating and conquering elevated blood pressure. Generally, recommendations are to attempt to lower high blood pressure through lifestyle modifications (see table 1.3) over a three- to six-month period. If this trial period is unsuccessful or initial blood pressures are greater than 160/100 mmHg, then medication should be added to the plan.

Table 1.3 **Lifestyle Modifications to Reduce and Control Blood Pressure**

Modification	Recommendation	Approximate reduction in systolic blood pressure
Weight loss	Maintain BMI from 18.5–24.9 kg/m²	5–20 mmHg
DASH diet	Make your diet high in vegetables and fruit and low in fat	8–14 mmHg
Reduced sodium	Eat 2.4 grams or less of sodium per day	2–8 mmHg
Physical activity	Exercise 30 minutes daily, most days of the week	4–9 mmHg
Moderate alcohol	Limit to one or two drinks daily	2–4 mmHg

Adapted from A.V. Chobanian, G.L. Bakris, H.R. Black, et al. 2003. "The seventh report of the Joint National Committee on Prevention, Detection, Evaluation, and Treatment of High Blood Pressure: the JNC 7 report." *Journal of the American Medical Association* 289: 2560-2572.

Taking the Time to Stay Healthy

A successful businessperson and company owner in his 40s, Jerry had the world by the tail. He worked hard to achieve what he had and knew no other way. A genuinely nice guy, he could become stressed out with the best of them. He had no time for himself and no time to exercise. When his blood pressure got higher, he saw his physician for a physical and casually mentioned an "odd" feeling in his chest. Many members of his family had heart disease, some at a young age, yet Jerry was too busy running his company and enjoying life to think the odd feeling was heart disease. When his doctor finally persuaded him to have it thoroughly checked out, he was so sure it was not heart related that he bet his doctor $10 that it wasn't. Jerry lost the $10 but gained his life back after his bypass surgery. Now he exercises, keeps his stress under control, and continues to enjoy life—only more so than before, as it was almost taken from him due to his own denial.

At this point it should be apparent that exercise should have a vital role in the treatment of high blood pressure, but it often is underemphasized in the management plan. As physicians we try to control what we can in the management of an illness, and the proper dispensing of medication allows us to do this. Unfortunately, we rely on medication far too often in the management of high blood pressure. We neglect to emphasize the importance of lifestyle management, such as beginning and maintaining an appropriate exercise program, losing weight, eating right, and doing a better job of managing stress.

Exercising to Affect Blood Pressure

Because of the increased demands placed on the body's systems during exercise, blood pressure must go up during exercise. In general, systolic blood pressure rises 8 to 12 mmHg for every metabolic equivalent (MET) above rest. One MET is the amount of oxygen used, or consumed, while at rest. An activity that is 2 METs requires twice the amount of oxygen, 3 METs requires three times as much, and so on. We will discuss METs in more detail in chapter 4. Because more blood flow is needed during exercise, the body should automatically reduce the level of resistance to blood flow within the blood vessels during exercise to meet this demand. Thus, *diastolic pressure should go down with exercise*. In some people with hypertension, the normal mechanism to lower diastolic pressure during exercise is faulty and diastolic pressure may rise.

Immediately after exercise, most people will experience a phenomenon referred to as *postexercise hypotension,* or a lowering of blood pressure. This can occur with an exercise interval as short as 10 minutes at low exercise intensity (about 40 percent of maximum heart rate). In general, a 5- to 7-mmHg reduction in blood pressure is present for up to 24 hours after exercise. Some researchers believe this is the basic mechanism for the reduction of blood pressure seen with programs of regular exercise. Furthermore, other researchers have found that the simple awareness of this phenomenon by people with hypertension helps to promote their adherence to their individual training program.

The optimum "dose" of exercise is 30 minutes of aerobic activity, which results in an increase in heart rate from 55 to 70 percent of maximum, on most days of the week. For most, the best aerobic activity will be walking; however, several other types of activities are also possible. Some form of strength and flexibility training would also benefit your overall program. Teaching you how to apply the optimum amount and type of exercise to lower your blood pressure is the main purpose of this book. More doctors and patients should view exercise in the same way that they view the use of medications; in other words, an exercise prescription would be an appropriate "drug" for many diseases.

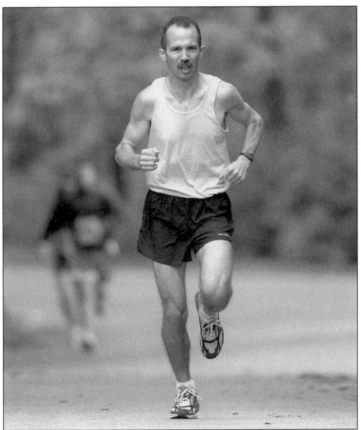

© Human Kinetics

Adherence to a regular exercise program can prolong and maximize the reduction in blood pressure that follows a single 10-minute bout of exercise.

The Exercise Prescription

▸ An endurance activity involving the majority of muscle groups

▸ Activity resulting in the heart rate increasing to 55 to 70 percent of maximum

▸ Done 30 continuous or accumulated minutes (such as 10 minutes on three occasions) per day

▸ Taken daily, in single or more frequent shorter doses

If you are starting a new exercise program, once you begin your program, it will take about 6 to 12 weeks to see the effects of exercise on your blood pressure. It will be a gradual effect. You will also notice that your blood pressure during exercise does not go up as much with the same intensity of exercise. Also, within about 2 to 3 weeks, you will notice that workouts become easier and that your progress is greatest during this time. After about 3 weeks, your new program will become a healthy habit, which will make it much easier to schedule into your day. On days you don't exercise, you will miss it. Weight loss generally begins during this time. Noticeable changes in strength and flexibility will become evident. Within about 6 weeks, you will look different and feel your clothes fit differently.

If you retake your resting blood pressure again between 6 and 12 weeks into your program, you will probably see a 5- to 10-mmHg reduction in both systolic and diastolic pressures. For those in the prehypertensive or stage 1 disease severity ranges, this will bring you into the ideal range. Congratulations and keep up the good work!

Establishing the Healthy Habit of Exercise for a Lifetime

At 95 years of age, Walter was a dapper dresser who walked one to two miles daily. His systolic pressures were consistently above 170; however, he was never treated for hypertension. When his doctor suggested a low-dose medication to try to lower his pressure, he reluctantly agreed. Within two weeks, he didn't like the idea of taking medications and stopped taking them. His pressure remained high but he continued walking daily. His pressure was still elevated on his 100th birthday. Moral of the story: Doctor, don't mess with someone who makes it to 95!

At this point, you have also significantly reduced your risk of heart disease, in some cases by almost 50 percent. You have significantly reduced your risk of stroke by a similar percentage. You have probably lost anywhere from 5 to 15 pounds, depending on which diet you are following.

You may prefer a fruit snack to baked goods or ice cream. You may have reduced or quit smoking. After all, good smokers are not good exercisers and vice versa. You may notice that things that used to really irritate you, or increase your anxiety, are less likely to do so. If you have made it to six weeks without a major musculoskeletal overuse injury, you also will be less likely to drop out of your exercise program because of a painful injury. Again, great job!

At some point in your management plan, your doctor may recommend medication to control your blood pressure. As we will discuss in later sections, there are medications that are better for active individuals. To be effective, medication should

- work by gradually reducing blood pressure to the ideal target range,
- be free of side effects that create other problems and discourage regular use, and
- be easy for you to remember to take—ideally, once daily.

Summary

Shouldn't everyone with high blood pressure be active? The answer is definitely yes! Unfortunately, not everyone gets that message and would rather rely on medication alone. But the potential of exercise to maintain healthy blood pressure levels is great, and in many cases it can be used instead of medication. An appropriate exercise plan added to healthy eating and, when necessary, medication, can give you the best results. This book shows you how to customize your exercise for this purpose, and you will be taking control of the management of your blood pressure and feeling better in many ways because of it.

WINNING THE BLOOD PRESSURE BATTLE

☐ Know the risk factors for hypertension and which ones you possess.

☐ Understand the workings of your heart and arteries; be familiar with terms such as *systolic pressure* and *diastolic pressure*.

☐ Be aware of the causes of elevated blood pressure and identify which ones you can prevent.

☐ Encourage yourself with the knowledge that blood pressure can be lowered through certain lifestyle modifications:

- Weight loss
- Physical activity and exercise
- Healthy eating habits such as low sodium, low fat, and high percentage of vegetables and fruits

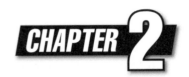

CHAPTER 2

CONQUERING HYPERTENSION WITH EXERCISE

Now that we've established that regular exercise has some benefit in reducing high blood pressure, it's time to determine what types of exercise will reduce pressure and how much exercise is right for you. We'll also discuss how you can build activity into your busy life. This chapter gives an overview of the three main modes of exercise that round out a complete exercise program—aerobic activity, strength training, and flexibility—and how they work to stabilize blood pressure. We will elaborate more on these modes in subsequent chapters, and specific programs and exercises will be detailed.

Choosing Exercise Modes

Unless you are an aerobics instructor or a mail carrier, you probably do not get enough activity in your day to lower your blood pressure without a program of regular exercise. Even if you have a very active occupation, do your job requirements include the amount of activity needed for lowering pressure? Does it allow you to adapt to increasing workloads over time? Does going to work every day lower your blood pressure? The answer for most of us would be no. Only a few of us have jobs that allow us to be active enough to maintain a lower blood pressure, have fewer side effects of hypertension, and live longer, more productive lives.

The secret seems to be the number of calories we burn. In an early report of the famous Harvard alumni study, all-cause mortality rates were one quarter to one third lower among male alumni expending 2,000 or more calories during exercise per week than among less active male alumni (Paffenbarger et al. 1986). Many subsequent long-term studies of large numbers of people have confirmed that individuals who are moderately active live longer. So, is the secret to a long life burning calories? Probably. It seems that in addition to other healthy lifestyle habits, and good genes, individuals who burn calories through activity will live longer.

When we say *active,* what do we mean? Most adults require between 1,500 and 2,500 calories daily to sustain normal function. What was found in these large studies of activity was that the individuals who lived longer expended 1,500 to 2,500 calories per week above that of the normal resting level. This means that on a daily basis, they did activities that cost the body about 200 to 300 extra calories, total. In other words, by doing something, anything, on a daily basis, that required the amount of energy contained in a small piece of chocolate cake or a regular-sized hamburger, you can live longer. If only the energy cost for us to eat the cake was the same as the calories in the cake, we would have it made.

Aerobic Activity

So, about how many calories would it take to make a cake and eat it? To prepare, bake, frost, and eat a cake requires about 100 calories, so you would probably need to make two or three cakes an hour in order to enjoy just one piece. On the other hand, if you walked to the bakery a mile away and took about 15 to 20 minutes to get there, you could sit down and enjoy the piece of cake without any caloric gain, as long as you walked back! In other words, a 2-mile walk in 30 to 40 minutes would burn about 250 to 300 calories.

In this example, a baker works hard to make cakes, but he burns only about 100 calories—a smaller amount than that burned in a brisk 30-minute walk. Why is this so? Because walking requires the use of many muscle groups, all of which must burn calories for fuel to sustain activity. The more muscles that are involved, the more fuel is needed. Walking faster or jogging requires even more fuel. Activity that requires a large percentage of muscle groups working at a moderate level of intensity is referred to as *aerobic activity. Aerobic* means that to burn calories the body requires oxygen delivery to the muscles.

Sprinting to the bakery, rather than walking or running, increases the muscles' demands for oxygen above the body's ability to supply it, so the energy production cannot be maintained. You can probably sprint for a minute or so, and then you have to slow down to allow your oxygen delivery system time to catch up. By that time, you will have burned only about 100 calories. This is why it's important to achieve an appropriate level of exercise intensity—too little and you won't burn enough calories, too much and you'll wear out too quickly.

Intensity

The easiest way to gauge aerobic exercise intensity is to measure your heart rate. In general, an activity that is aerobic will result in a heart rate increase of about 40 to 70 beats above resting heart rate, or 60 to 85 percent of your maximum heart rate (maximum heart rate is discussed further in chapter 4). Intense activities, such as running up several flights of stairs quickly or sprinting, increase the heart rate above 85 percent of maximum and far exceed the body's ability to deliver oxygen. Associated with this increase is heavy breathing to the point of feeling short of breath and a burning sensation in the muscles. In order to recover, your activity level needs to slow enough to drop your heart rate below 60 percent. Unless you can continually maintain this form of torture (referred to as *interval training* and discussed later in the book), doesn't it make sense to find a pace of activity that allows the heart rate to fall within the 60 to 85 percent range? This would allow you to maintain the appropriate level of activity for longer than a minute or so without significant discomfort.

If some is good, more is better, right? Not necessarily! This is an error many people make when planning an exercise program. If the activity you have chosen to burn off those pounds is too intense, you will not meet your goal because you cannot sustain the beneficial level of activity. The ideal amount of activity intensity for blood pressure control should cause your heart rate to rise to 40 to 70 beats above resting, or to 60 to 85 percent of its maximum.

Pump Function

So how does aerobic exercise affect blood pressure? Anyone who exercises, or has run up a flight or two of stairs occasionally, knows that exercise causes your heart rate and breathing rate to go up. These increases meet the demands for more oxygen at the level of the working muscles. To get the oxygen where it is needed, we breathe faster, allowing more oxygen to pass into the bloodstream per minute. In order to get the oxygenated blood to the muscle faster, our heart rate speeds up and our blood pressure rises, usually about 8 to 12 mmHg with each MET, or unit of energy expenditure above resting (Naughton and Haider 1973). The exercising pressure rises due to the increase in heart rate and in the force of each heart contraction. In other words, the heart pumps faster and stronger. In medical terms, the *stroke volume,* or amount of blood pumped out from the heart with each heartbeat, increases. The extra work increases the energy demands for the heart itself, so it is absolutely essential that blood flow to the heart muscle not be obstructed in any way, or else the pump does not function well. Individuals with coronary artery disease, or blockage in the arteries leading to the heart muscle, may have limited pump function caused by this obstruction.

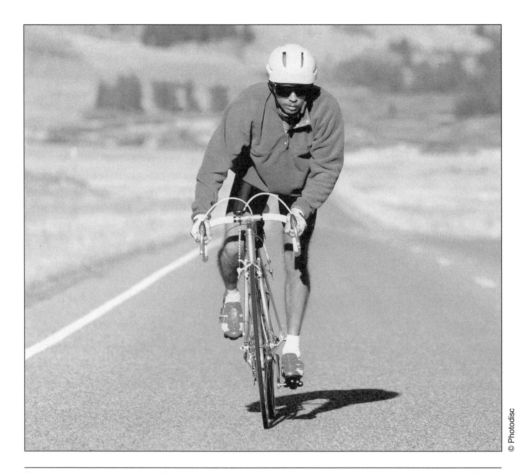

Exercise is considered aerobic if it uses multiple muscle groups and requires oxygen delivery to the muscles so they can burn calories for fuel.

Assuming the demand of blood flow to the heart muscle is being adequately supplied and the heart is functioning at maximum efficiency, the blood flow to the rest of the body goes up dramatically. Resting *cardiac output,* or the amount of blood pumped from the heart in one minute, is normally 5 liters per minute for men and slightly less for women. As exercise intensity increases, cardiac output increases rapidly to meet the body's demands and levels off as the demand is achieved. If the demand for more oxygenated blood flow increases because the physical task becomes harder, cardiac output again increases and levels off when the demand is met or the individual's maximum cardiac output, generally 20 to 25 liters per minute, is reached.

Total Peripheral Resistance and Oxygen Delivery

In order for the blood to be efficiently delivered to the exercising muscles, the resistance in the pipelines needs to be lowered. As exercise intensity increases, the body's arterial pipelines widen to allow more unobstructed flow to the active muscles. In addition to the widening of the arteries to working muscles, arterial flow to other inactive tissues in the body is decreased or shunted away from where extra blood flow is not needed at that moment. This process is achieved by involuntary contraction of smooth muscle within the blood vessel. An increase in the smooth muscle contraction results in decreased blood flow past the contraction. The sum total of resistance or *total peripheral resistance (TPR)* to blood flow generally decreases during exercise.

An individual's maximum exercise or work capacity is rarely limited by the body's ability to supply blood to exercising muscle. If this is the case, why can't we all run marathons or complete the Tour de France at blazing speeds? The limiting factor is in the muscle itself, not the blood supply. Similar to the old adage of "you can lead a horse to water, but you can't make him drink," well-oxygenated blood reaches and passes into the muscle very well, but the muscle has only so much metabolic machinery to process the delivered oxygen. The amount of machinery depends on several factors. Most influential is how much machinery our parents placed into our muscles—genetics plays a major role in exercise utilization of oxygen. Another influence is our level of fitness. A fit individual has more oxygen-utilization machinery present in the muscle than a less fit individual. An individual's maximum oxygen utilization capacity for all muscles is collectively referred to as *maximum oxygen uptake* or $\dot{V}O_2max$.

The elevation in exercising blood pressure is the mathematical (and functional) product of the cardiac output (how hard the pump is pumping) and the total peripheral resistance (how much resistance to flow is in the pipes leading from the pump). The increase in blood pressure during exercise is not only normal but is also essential for meeting the demands of the working muscles. Individuals with high resting blood pressure will have higher exercising blood pressure. As long as the systolic pressure is not excessive (greater than 220 mmHg), this elevation is not harmful to pressure-sensitive tissues such as the brain, heart, eyes, or kidneys.

With regular exercise, several beneficial changes occur. Cardiac output generally increases slightly for a given amount of work because the stroke volume increases. The heart contraction becomes stronger and more blood is returned to the heart, allowing it to pump a higher volume of blood with each stroke. The total peripheral resistance generally decreases to allow more efficient delivery of oxygenated blood to working muscles. This acute decrease in TPR carries over into the postexercise period, resulting in lower systolic and diastolic blood pressure—a phenomenon exercise scientists refer to as *postexercise hypotension* (PEH), which may last up to 22 hours after a workout (Ronda et al. 2002). It is currently unclear what is the exact contribution of acute exercise to PEH; PEH has been reported to occur following as little as 3 minutes of exercise (Kraul et al. 1966) and at low exercise intensity (Pescatello et al. 1991). Regardless of the amount of exercise, PEH was greater in those who started off with a higher resting pressure. Therefore, the body's natural response to lowering blood pressure with exercise training seems to work best for those who need it the most—those with hypertension (American College of Sports Medicine 2004).

Other mechanisms are at work that result in elevated blood pressure. TPR is lower at rest in those who are more fit. Currently, it is thought that TPR is regulated primarily by the brain and autonomic nervous system. Epinephrine (adrenaline) and cortisol, the body's primary stress hormone, both go up when we are acutely stressed. An elevation in epinephrine increases TPR, resulting in an increase in both systolic and diastolic blood pressure. Regular exposure to stress results in more frequently elevated epinephrine and higher levels of cortisol. Thus with increased stress, epinephrine and cortisol levels are elevated, resulting in higher TPR and, thus, higher blood pressure. When stress is lessened, the reverse occurs.

Other factors can increase TPR. Individuals with peripheral vascular disease, for example, have significant plaque buildup in the major arteries of the body, which may increase peripheral resistance and potentially limit blood flow to exercising muscle. Obesity also raises TPR, which is one of the main reasons obesity is associated with hypertension. Although excess adipose tissue (fat) and plaque buildup inside the arteries tend to occur together, it is the extra adipose tissue that increases TPR by squeezing the arteries from the outside.

With regular exercise, TPR is reduced resulting in lower blood pressure; the primary effect seems to be a "chronic" state of PEH. The bottom line, which is very well supported by the scientific literature, is that *individuals who participate in a regular aerobic exercise program can reduce their blood pressure, and this effect is generally greater for those who were hypertensive before beginning training.* In order to be fit, and to reduce your blood pressure, follow the FITT program detailed in the following sidebar.

Becoming FITT

The acronym FITT is a handy way to remember four components that make up a comprehensive fitness program—frequency, intensity, time, and type. Here we describe them and their optimal amounts. These terms are also defined more fully on pages 25-26.

Frequency: Exercise every day of the week, if possible, or at least most days.

Intensity: Work at moderate intensity, 40 to 60 percent of maximal capacity.

Time: Get at least 30 minutes of continuous or accumulated physical activity per day.

Type: Try to do primarily endurance physical activity (for example, walking, running, cycling, rowing, swimming, or heavy gardening and yard work) supplemented by resistance exercise.

Result: Seek to burn about 300 calories per workout and reduce postexercise resting blood pressure 5 to 7 mmHg (ACSM 2004).

Strength Training

Remember the story of Milo, the boy who lifted a calf each day and grew stronger as the calf grew heavier? This is one of the best analogies to explain the *overload principle* of strength training. As workload increases, our muscular system adapts to the increased load by several mechanisms. The ability to lift heavier weights more than likely occurs because of the coordination between the nervous and muscular systems. This adaptation or improved functional coordination occurs by both voluntary and involuntary methods. The most visible of these changes is increased muscle tone. Tone is merely the body's method of turning on the neuromuscular "switch" to a muscle or group of muscles. With repetition of an exercise or sports skill, your body's coordination between the nervous system and the muscles used in the activity becomes more efficient. With practice, the activity becomes easier, because these two systems are better coordinated, and best yet the improved coordination is done without a lot of thought. The increase in tone is associated with an increase in muscle size. The size increase allows muscle groups the ability to maintain a contraction with the movement of a heavier load. As you may be aware, some individuals are blessed with the ability to adapt to increasing loads with larger muscles. Again, this is most likely a genetic influence. Unfortunately, some will try to speed up the training process or attempt to make up for genetics through the use of medications such as anabolic steroids, growth hormones, or other ergogenic aids. If you use these medications, your risk of developing and worsening blood pressure and many other conditions such as heart disease, vascular disease, and some forms of cancer is far greater.

In the past, people with high blood pressure were told to avoid strength training because it was thought that it may increase blood pressure. We now know that this is not true and confuses the concepts of strength training with the sport of weightlifting. In a large analysis of several studies on resistance training, Kelley and Kelley (2000) reported a systolic and diastolic blood pressure reduction of 3 mmHg, or 2 to 4 percent, for those with normal pressures and with hypertension. Although these changes are not as great as what would be expected with aerobic training, combining resistance and aerobic training results in an additive effect on blood pressure reduction.

Increased muscular strength results in improved movement efficiency, increased power, and better neuromuscular coordination. All of these effects contribute to more efficient movement and, more than likely, to the lower resting blood pressure associated with training. Other potential factors include increased capillary density in growing muscles, which helps lower total peripheral resistance (TPR). Similar to aerobic training, resistance training can also lower stress hormones, which can in turn lower TPR.

All of us, from the young to the very old, can benefit from some form of strength training. The first mental hurdle for some is to realize that

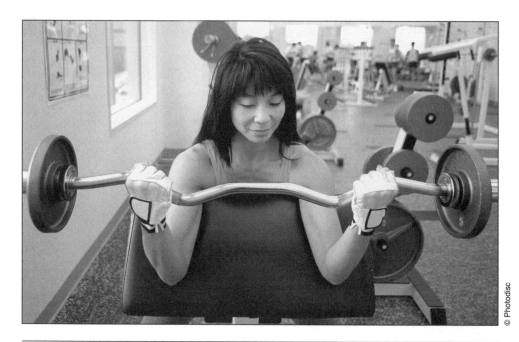

When proper technique is used, strength training contributes to lower resting blood pressure, and you benefit from the many advantages of having stronger, more efficient muscles.

strength training should not be confused with the sport of weightlifting. The goal in strength training is not to be able to lift a lot at one time but to be able to adapt to move, lift, and do other activities with increased efficiency. There are several safe and effective ways of including strength training in your regular exercise routine.

Isometrics, made famous by Charles Atlas in the 1950s, is the static contraction of a muscle, usually to its maximum contracted force, without movement of the limb involved in the contraction. Perhaps the best practical example of isometric contraction (often referred to as *static exercise*) is when you try very hard to lift an object that is too heavy. The muscles contract, the maximum force is applied, yet you and the object do not move. In the past, measurements of blood pressure during isometric contractions were reported to be extremely high and potentially dangerous for those who already had hypertension. But those studies have been repeated in recent years with different results: pressure measurements were not as high. In fact, current research indicates that static strength exercise is not only safer than previously reported but is also beneficial in reducing resting diastolic blood pressure in those with hypertension by as much as 5 mmHg. Because there are so few studies in this area, the evidence to support incorporating static exercise into a training program is promising, but not as overwhelming as the evidence for incorporating aerobic and resistance training into your program. This book will show you how to put together a strength-training program that will help you, not hurt you.

Flexibility Training

Perhaps the fastest-growing form of training is in the area of flexibility. Yoga, Pilates, and core training are all forms of training that combine some low-intensity aerobics with stretching. If done correctly, flexibility training improves the stretching capabilities of the muscles and tendons across the joints. This generally allows us to move more fluidly, without stiffness and generally without pain.

Currently, scientists are debating whether flexibility reduces the risk of injury, as has been thought for several years. People who regularly do some form of appropriate flexibility training report that they feel better, move better, and have less painful stiffness than those who don't stretch regularly. In addition to these improvements, those who perform flexibility training regularly have an improved sense of well-being and report managing stress better. Another nice effect of flexibility training is that it may help reduce any stress-induced cause of blood pressure elevation in those with hypertension.

Yoga has been used for centuries as a form of stress management. Newer forms of movement to improve balance, flexibility, and strength, such as Nia, Pilates, and core strength training, efficiently combine activities that are ideal for those with elevated blood pressure. Therefore, our goal to improve the efficiency of your very tightly scheduled exercise program is to include flexibility training to reduce the tension in your mind and muscles. In later chapters we will introduce several flexibility training techniques.

Identifying Exercise Components and Principles

Within the three main modes of exercise are different types of exercise: for example, aerobic exercise types include running, walking, swimming, and cycling. Whichever type you choose, you will need to calculate some important numbers when putting together a program. These include frequency, intensity, amount of time, and type of exercise. You'll remember these from the sidebar on FITT (page 22). Other principles of exercise that will ensure improvement are *overload, progression,* and *specificity.* These are considered the specific ingredients of an exercise program. We will go into more detail on how to figure these components in chapters 4, 5, and 6, but this section gives you an overview of these elements.

Frequency refers to how often during a given week you work out. Some form of exercise most days of the week, or daily, is ideal.

Intensity refers to how difficult or easy a given workout feels. High-intensity exercise approaches your maximum effort, while low-intensity exercise is felt to be easy. There are several ways to measure exercise intensity: the heart rate required, the amount of oxygen needed, and the amount of calories burned. Perhaps the easiest way to determine exercise intensity is the talk test. If you cannot easily carry on a conversation while you are exercising, then the intensity is probably high. If you can (and you are not breathing harder or faster), the exercise intensity is probably low. Ideally, the amount of exercise intensity should be moderate, about 40 to 60 percent of maximum effort.

Time refers to the amount of minutes of continuous exercise done in a workout. The ideal amount of continuous exercise per workout should be at least 30 minutes.

Type refers to the exercise task at hand: walking, running, or cycling, for example. The ideal type of exercise should work many muscle groups and be primarily an endurance activity supplemented by resistance exercise.

Overload describes a principle stating that in order to become more fit, the body must be stressed above the status quo. If you follow the FITT plan, your body will be appropriately stressed above the status quo, resulting in the physical adaptations described in the previous sections.

Progression describes the gradual increase in frequency, intensity, and time needed for the body to become more fit. The amount of work required for the body to adapt varies by individual. Initially, the amount of increase in the program, or overload, should be gradual. This gradual increase in overload is referred to as the program's progression. Once the many systems adapt to the amount of overload, the amount of overload must gradually increase, or else no additional adaptation will take place. The amount of exercise progression is felt by many exercise professionals to be more art than science.

Specificity refers to a basic training principle stating that the body will adapt only to the demands of the exercise program being done for training. In other words, endurance training improves endurance, not sprinting ability; strength training improves strength, not flexibility; hitting a baseball improves ability to hit a baseball, not shoot a basket. Although there is occasional overlap of a specific training routine affecting other skills and tasks, in general, if you want to improve a skill or system, repeat that skill or train that system.

Maintaining an Active Lifestyle and Having Fun With Fitness

In addition to maintaining an exercise program, it is important to adopt an active lifestyle. Simple daily activities such as taking the stairs instead of the elevator, parking farther away from the entrance of a store, and choosing hobbies that promote movement and physical activity all will contribute positively to your blood pressure reduction program. Taking public transportation, cycling, and walking when you can tend to increase activity more than driving your own vehicle where you want to go.

Unfortunately, it is often difficult to maintain an active lifestyle when time is at a premium. Nowhere is this reality more evident than in our daily grind back and forth to work. One of the reasons Houston was selected as a "fat city" was the amount of commute time, which takes away from daily exercise time. Certainly, our sprawling cities increase the amount of time we are behind the wheel. The added commute time requirement certainly forces us to be more creative in choosing when and where to exercise. If your schedule is flexible, avoiding the typical daily rush hours can add time to your day. Exercise before or after work at a facility on or near your worksite to avoid at least one leg of the daily rush hours. Break times and lunch hours are an ideal time to add a 20-minute walk to your day.

Enjoy it; play at it. Fitness for the sake of fitness is boring for some. The drudgery of going to the gym every day soon after making those New Year's resolutions has been the undoing of many a good intention. To be successful in your fitness goals, exercise needs to become something you really enjoy doing. Children play every day because they enjoy it. Couldn't

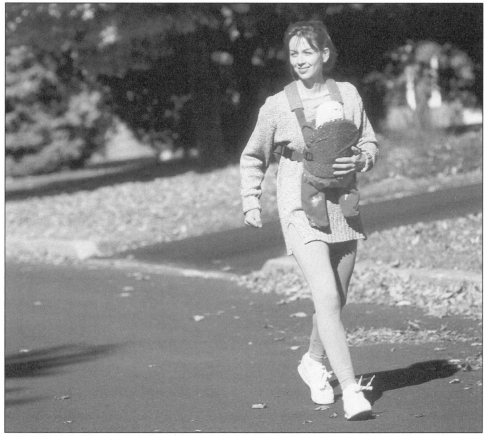

© Comstock

Combining exercise with spending time with your children can be a creative way to fit physical activity into a busy life.

we adapt the same idea with exercise? Whether it is the new bike we love to ride, our workout buddies we enjoy spending time with, or the idea of trying to improve each aspect of our game, all these features of a regular fitness program will make it fun. When exercise becomes play, it automatically becomes a priority in our daily schedule.

Even the most fun game can become boring, so it is also important to vary activity in order for it to remain fun. Varying activities helps your body to train in different ways and your mind to continue to enjoy what you are doing. If you belong to a gym, don't go to the same class five times a week and ignore the lap pool. Devout runners and cyclists should vary their route, pace, and distance. Variety will help you maintain your interests and, ultimately, your health.

Don't forget who you play with. A common method of improving exercise adherence and making the workout more fun is to involve a training partner or two. The attraction of team sports for many is the opportunity for regular social interaction. Going at it alone is fine for some; however, most who begin a new program of exercise are more likely to stay with it if they have very good social support from family or friends. Families committed to the fitness of individual members should consider exercising together.

Turning Fun Into Exercise

Just for fun, I wore my heart rate monitor during a couple hours of sledding with my boys. I was surprised to see that over 90 minutes of fun, my heart rate averaged within my training range of 130 to 158 and peaked at 170! Sledding down our small hill and walking back up the hill burned about 700 calories over 90 minutes. Certainly, other kid-friendly activities such as in-line skating, hiking, swimming, and cycling are good options. Don't underestimate the fitness value of playing with your kids regularly.

Summary

Whatever you decide to do, do it and have fun. Be flexible with your schedule and choice of activities. Choosing activities you really enjoy will make you more likely to stick with it. Be creative. In the management of hypertension, exercise is often as good as a pill, but any good physician knows the patient needs to be evaluated before the right pill can be given. The strenuous-yardwork pill doesn't work well for the city townhouse dweller, and the running-an-8-minute-mile pill doesn't work well for the individual getting off the couch for the first time. I think you get the picture—we need to decide which pill is best for you.

CONQUERING HYPERTENSION WITH EXERCISE

☐ Learn how many calories of energy expenditure are required to gain health benefits of exercise.

☐ Find out how each mode of exercise (aerobic, resistance, and flexibility) affects blood pressure.

☐ Consider important exercise variables:

- Frequency
- Intensity
- Amount of time
- Type

☐ Remember the exercise principles of overload, progression, and specificity.

☐ Brainstorm ways to fit more physical activity into your daily life.

CHAPTER 3

ASSESSING YOUR FITNESS LEVEL

To maximize the potential of exercise to reduce high blood pressure, improve your fitness level, and yield other health benefits, you need to determine your current fitness level and create an exercise program that fits your specific needs and encourages improvement. Completing some assessment tests and measurements and comparing your results to fitness norms is a helpful way to discover your fitness level. This chapter gives instructions on such tests—specifically, for aerobic fitness, strength, and flexibility—and shows you how to interpret the results. But first, let's talk about another important task: seeing your doctor to get a thorough examination and discuss any precautions you should take with exercise.

Obtaining a Physician's Exam

An annual exam by a physician who knows you well is the most valuable diagnostic tool at your disposal. An established relationship with your family doctor is essential for optimal care of high blood pressure and other chronic health problems. In general, for someone with new or chronic hypertension, an annual physical exam should focus on identifying and controlling risk factors associated with worsening blood pressure or heart disease, evaluating possible "targeted" organ damage caused by high blood pressure, and identifying potential coronary vascular disease (CVD) complications.

Annual exams should build on an established base of your medical history (previous health issues) and family history and include a current review of any active or recent symptoms. As a complement to this symptom review, you and your physician should examine all systems completely to uncover any potential concerns that may exist but appear to you not to be related. The annual exam is also a good time to update any health maintenance issues such as immunizations, positive and negative health habits, and the influence of the environment and community on your current health.

A complete exam from head to toe, and everything in between, is usually done; however, your physician may elect to exclude certain portions of the exam based on your health history. In most cases, though, the complete exam will be done. Almost every system is affected by high blood pressure, so plan on having an eye exam, thorough heart exam, abdominal and rectal exam, and an exam of the limbs, spine, and joints—especially if you are active. Those who spend a great deal of time outdoors or who have a fair complexion should have a head-to-toe skin exam to detect any possible skin cancers. Women should have a breast exam annually after age 30 and a pelvic exam. Men should plan on a prostate exam annually after age 40.

A complete battery of blood tests is important. A complete blood cell count, electrolyte levels, kidney and liver functions, glucose and cholesterol studies, and a urinalysis to look for traces of hidden blood or elevated protein levels are usually all that are needed. Additional blood tests, such as thyroid studies, additional kidney function tests, and other hormonal tests, may be done during the initial exam to look for rare secondary causes of hypertension. If your physician elects not to do these additional tests during your initial exam, do not feel as if you're getting an incomplete evaluation. These secondary causes are so rare that most physicians will elect to do the tests only if you have a difficult time regulating your pressure with multiple interventions. If you are found to have one of these rare secondary causes, your physician will put you on a regular schedule for monitoring this condition, which may include blood, urine, or other imaging tests.

Some other tests your doctor may choose to run include a stress test to determine functional aerobic capacity, a nuclear imaging stress test to check blood flow and arteries, or other tests to measure cardiac health.

If you are starting a new exercise program, it's a good idea to complete a questionnaire called the Physical Activity Readiness Questionnaire (PAR-Q) to determine whether you need to see your doctor specifically about beginning exercise. This form is shown in figure 3.1.

Evaluating Aerobic Capacity

Once your doctor has cleared you to exercise, it's time to determine how fit you are and where to begin, or how to adjust your program if you've already been exercising. Your first step in the lifelong fitness journey will be to estimate your $\dot{V}O_2$max, or how effectively your body uses the oxygen you breathe in. $\dot{V}O_2$max is reported in several forms, the most common being in units of milliliters of oxygen used per kilogram of body weight per

Physical Activity Readiness
Questionnaire - PAR-Q
(revised 2002)

PAR-Q & YOU

(A Questionnaire for People Aged 15 to 69)

Regular physical activity is fun and healthy, and increasingly more people are starting to become more active every day. Being more active is very safe for most people. However, some people should check with their doctor before they start becoming much more physically active.

If you are planning to become much more physically active than you are now, start by answering the seven questions in the box below. If you are between the ages of 15 and 69, the PAR-Q will tell you if you should check with your doctor before you start. If you are over 69 years of age, and you are not used to being very active, check with your doctor.

Common sense is your best guide when you answer these questions. Please read the questions carefully and answer each one honestly: check YES or NO.

YES	NO		
☐	☐	1.	Has your doctor ever said that you have a heart condition <u>and</u> that you should only do physical activity recommended by a doctor?
☐	☐	2.	Do you feel pain in your chest when you do physical activity?
☐	☐	3.	In the past month, have you had chest pain when you were not doing physical activity?
☐	☐	4.	Do you lose your balance because of dizziness or do you ever lose consciousness?
☐	☐	5.	Do you have a bone or joint problem (for example, back, knee or hip) that could be made worse by a change in your physical activity?
☐	☐	6.	Is your doctor currently prescribing drugs (for example, water pills) for your blood pressure or heart condition?
☐	☐	7.	Do you know of <u>any other reason</u> why you should not do physical activity?

If

you

answered

YES to one or more questions

Talk with your doctor by phone or in person BEFORE you start becoming much more physically active or BEFORE you have a fitness appraisal. Tell your doctor about the PAR-Q and which questions you answered YES.

- You may be able to do any activity you want — as long as you start slowly and build up gradually. Or, you may need to restrict your activities to those which are safe for you. Talk with your doctor about the kinds of activities you wish to participate in and follow his/her advice.
- Find out which community programs are safe and helpful for you.

NO to all questions

If you answered NO honestly to <u>all</u> PAR-Q questions, you can be reasonably sure that you can:

- start becoming much more physically active – begin slowly and build up gradually. This is the safest and easiest way to go.
- take part in a fitness appraisal – this is an excellent way to determine your basic fitness so that you can plan the best way for you to live actively. It is also highly recommended that you have your blood pressure evaluated. If your reading is over 144/94, talk with your doctor before you start becoming much more physically active.

DELAY BECOMING MUCH MORE ACTIVE:

- if you are not feeling well because of a temporary illness such as a cold or a fever – wait until you feel better; or
- if you are or may be pregnant – talk to your doctor before you start becoming more active.

PLEASE NOTE: If your health changes so that you then answer YES to any of the above questions, tell your fitness or health professional. Ask whether you should change your physical activity plan.

<u>Informed Use of the PAR-Q</u>: The Canadian Society for Exercise Physiology, Health Canada, and their agents assume no liability for persons who undertake physical activity, and if in doubt after completing this questionnaire, consult your doctor prior to physical activity.

No changes permitted. You are encouraged to photocopy the PAR-Q but only if you use the entire form.

NOTE: If the PAR-Q is being given to a person before he or she participates in a physical activity program or a fitness appraisal, this section may be used for legal or administrative purposes.

"I have read, understood and completed this questionnaire. Any questions I had were answered to my full satisfaction."

NAME _____

SIGNATURE _____ DATE _____

SIGNATURE OF PARENT _____ WITNESS _____
or GUARDIAN (for participants under the age of majority)

Note: This physical activity clearance is valid for a maximum of 12 months from the date it is completed and becomes invalid if your condition changes so that you would answer YES to any of the seven questions.

CSEP
SCPE © Canadian Society for Exercise Physiology   Supported by: ▮✦ Health Canada Santé Canada

continued on other side...

(continued)

Figure 3.1 Physical Activity Readiness Questionnaire (PAR-Q).

From *Action Plan for High Blood Pressure* by Jon G. Divine, 2006, Champaign, IL: Human Kinetics.

Source: Physical Activity Readiness Questionnaire (PAR-Q) © 2002. Reproduced with permission from the Canadian Society for Exercise Physiology. www.csep.ca/forms.asp

...continued from other side

PAR-Q & YOU

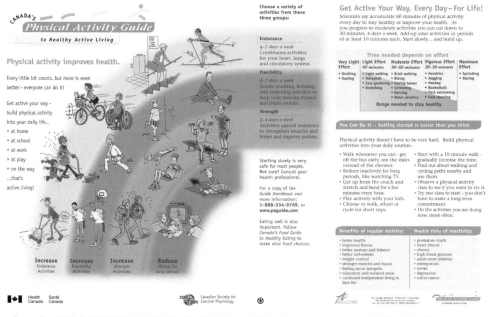

Source: *Canada's Physical Activity Guide to Healthy Active Living*, Health Canada, 1998 http://www.hc-sc.gc.ca/hppb/paguide/pdf/guideEng.pdf
© Reproduced with permission from the Minister of Public Works and Government Services Canada, 2002.

FITNESS AND HEALTH PROFESSIONALS MAY BE INTERESTED IN THE INFORMATION BELOW:

The following companion forms are available for doctors' use by contacting the Canadian Society for Exercise Physiology (address below):

The **Physical Activity Readiness Medical Examination (PARmed-X)** – to be used by doctors with people who answer YES to one or more questions on the PAR-Q.

The **Physical Activity Readiness Medical Examination for Pregnancy (PARmed-X for Pregnancy)** – to be used by doctors with pregnant patients who wish to become more active.

References:
Arraix, G.A., Wigle, D.T., Mao, Y. (1992). Risk Assessment of Physical Activity and Physical Fitness in the Canada Health Survey
    Follow-Up Study. **J. Clin. Epidemiol.** 45:4 419-428.
Mottola, M., Wolfe, L.A. (1994). Active Living and Pregnancy, In: A. Quinney, L. Gauvin, T. Wall (eds.), **Toward Active Living: Proceedings of the International**
    Conference on Physical Activity, Fitness and Health. Champaign, IL: Human Kinetics.
PAR-Q Validation Report, British Columbia Ministry of Health, 1978.
Thomas, S., Reading, J., Shephard, R.J. (1992). Revision of the Physical Activity Readiness Questionnaire (PAR-Q). **Can. J. Spt. Sci.** 17:4 338-345.

To order multiple printed copies of the PAR-Q, please contact the:

Canadian Society for Exercise Physiology
202-185 Somerset Street West
Ottawa, ON K2P 0J2
Tel. 1-877-651-3755 • FAX (613) 234-3565
Online: www.csep.ca

The original PAR-Q was developed by the British Columbia Ministry of Health. It has been revised by an Expert Advisory Committee of the Canadian Society for Exercise Physiology chaired by Dr. N. Gledhill (2002).

Disponible en français sous le titre «Questionnaire sur l'aptitude à l'activité physique - Q-AAP (revisé 2002)».

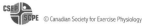 © Canadian Society for Exercise Physiology   Supported by: Health Canada   Santé Canada

---

Figure 3.1 *(continued)*

From *Action Plan for High Blood Pressure* by Jon G. Divine, 2006, Champaign, IL: Human Kinetics.

Source: Physical Activity Readiness Questionnaire (PAR-Q) © 2002. Reproduced with permission from the Canadian Society for Exercise Physiology. www.csep.ca/forms.asp

minute (ml/kg/min) or in metabolic equivalents (METs), which is the $\dot{V}O_2$ in ml/kg/min divided by 3.5. If you do a stress test or a monitored fitness test, the test technician should be able to provide these individualized numbers for you to use. Most people, however, do not have easy access to a monitored fitness test, so this chapter shows you ways to test yourself. Also, an assessment sheet is provided that you can use to record your scores (pages 51-52).

These will be important numbers for you to know about yourself because they will be used in later chapters to determine how much exercise to do and to measure your progress as you continue in your program. After your blood pressure values, $\dot{V}O_2$max is the next most important value for you in your quest to improve both your blood pressure and fitness.

One way to measure $\dot{V}O_2$max on your own is to take the Rockport 1-Mile Walk Test (see page 37), which identifies your fitness level based on how quickly you cover a given distance either walking or jogging. If you'd rather cycle, many fitness facilities have computerized stationary cycles that will easily estimate your $\dot{V}O_2$max based on your age, gender, and how well your heart performs on a built-in test. Some field tests will give a prediction of $\dot{V}O_2$max or METs as a measure of functional capacity (fitness); these values are then used to determine the relative intensity of how hard you need to exercise.

Table 3.1 shows you how your $\dot{V}O_2$max score stacks up against those of others of your age and gender. This information also serves as the basis for determining where you should start your exercise program. Once you have located your $\dot{V}O_2$max score in table 3.1, compare your score to the following breakdown of fitness levels: the 70th to 90th percentiles correspond to a high fitness level, the 40th to 60th to a medium fitness level, and the 10th to 30th to a low fitness level. The results from your aerobic fitness test and your level should be added to your individual assessment sheet (pages 51-52). In chapter 4 you will find beginning fitness programs for walking, running, cycling, and swimming that correspond to your fitness level; you will choose one to use for the aerobic portion of your exercise program. After 6 to 12 weeks you will need to reassess your fitness levels, which will most likely bump you up into a different level for your adjusted fitness program.

Just as you are determining your aerobic fitness level, you will determine your strength and flexibility levels later in this chapter. It is important to determine each of these three levels: aerobic fitness, strength, and flexibility. If you have a relatively low aerobic fitness score and a high strength score, for example, you would create a relatively easy aerobic program and a more challenging strength program. Each portion of your new fitness program is different, so if you are at one level for aerobics and another for strength or flexibility, you should begin your program based on the individual component's level. One level, just like one size, does not fit all.

Table 3.1 Aerobic Fitness Norms ($\dot{V}O_2max$)

Percentile	Age				
	20–29	30–39	40–49	50–59	Over 60
Men					
90	51.4	50.4	48.2	45.3	42.5
80	48.2	46.8	44.1	41.0	38.1
70	46.8	44.6	41.8	38.5	35.3
60	44.2	42.4	39.9	36.7	33.6
50	42.5	41.0	38.1	35.2	31.8
40	41.0	38.9	36.7	33.8	30.2
30	39.5	37.4	35.1	32.3	28.7
20	37.1	35.4	33.0	30.2	26.5
10	34.5	32.5	30.9	28.0	23.1
Women					
90	44.2	41.0	39.5	35.2	35.2
80	41.0	38.6	36.3	32.3	31.2
70	38.1	36.7	33.8	30.9	29.4
60	36.7	34.6	32.3	29.4	27.2
50	35.2	33.8	30.9	28.2	25.8
40	33.8	32.3	29.5	26.9	24.5
30	32.3	30.5	28.3	25.5	23.8
20	30.6	28.7	26.5	24.3	22.8
10	28.4	26.5	25.1	22.3	20.8

Reprinted, by permission, from American College of Sports Medicine (ACSM), 2000, *ACSM's guidelines for exercise testing and prescription,* 6th ed. (Baltimore, MD: Lippincott, Williams & Wilkins), 77.

Rockport 1-Mile Walk Test

One of the easiest ways to determine your fitness level is the Rockport 1-Mile Walk Test. All you need is a watch, a scale, a calculator, and a measured 1-mile route. If you live near a high school or college track, four times around (on the inside lanes) is 1 mile. Here's what you do:

- Weigh yourself before going to the track.
- Go to the track and walk a mile as fast as you can, timing yourself.
- At the end of the mile, before you take your victory lap, check your walk time in minutes and seconds.
- Then immediately take your pulse for 10 seconds.
- Write down your walk time and pulse.

Once you can get to a calculator, enter the numbers into the following equation:

$$\dot{V}O_2max = 132.853 - (0.0769 \times weight\ [lb]) - (0.3877 \times age\ [yr]) + (6.315 \times 0\ [females]\ or\ 1\ [males]) - (3.2649 \times time\ [min]) - (0.1565 \times HR)$$

Now you will have an accurate estimate of your $\dot{V}O_2max$ in ml/kg/min. What do you do with this number? We will use it later, so write it down somewhere. If you don't want to figure the calculation yourself, several Web sites will allow you to plug in your Rockport test values and instantly give you your $\dot{V}O_2max$ in units you can later use. These sites include the following:

- www.rockport.com/scripts/cgiip.exe/WService=rkptlatin1/10_walkingtest.html
- www.brianmac.demon.co.uk/rockport.htm
- www.exrx.net/Calculators/Rockport.html

Stationary Cycle Tests

Many health and fitness clubs have computer-controlled stationary cycles that will calculate your $\dot{V}O_2max$ while you work out. The instructions vary by bike manufacturer. All will ask you to begin to cycle at a comfortable pedaling rate (measured in revolutions per minute, or RPM) with an easy initial resistance. At some point you will be asked to enter your gender, age, and heart rate following an easy initial workload. The second stage will automatically increase to a harder workload while you maintain the same RPM. You will then need to enter a second heart rate for the work done at the higher workload. The computer will then calculate your $\dot{V}O_2max$ based on your inputs. Most of the results calculated are reliable and can be used to test your starting fitness level and repeated to monitor your progress. This option certainly can be appealing to those who don't trust their math skills!

Assessing Muscular Strength

Another important component of a well-rounded exercise program is the addition of resistance training to your aerobic training program. Just as in the aerobic program, it is important to obtain a baseline of your current strength ability in order to individualize your training program. Determining the correct amount of resistance to use is important so that you train efficiently: not too easy (which will not provide necessary overload and increase strength) and not too hard (which can result in easy fatigue and possible injury).

Two strength assessment tests, the one-repetition maximum bench press and leg press tests, can be done at most fitness clubs. Most clubs have resistance training equipment that will allow you to safely test your strength and then use the same equipment as part of your resistance training workout. If you are unsure how to properly use the resistance equipment or if it's your first time using a piece of exercise equipment, always ask for expert help and instruction from one of the fitness specialists in your club or gym.

An important tip to remember for any form of resistance training or testing is to perform each repetition properly. Do not alter form to lift a heavier weight, as this increases your risk of injury. It is also important to breathe correctly during all lifting activities: Inhale while lowering the weight and exhale while raising it, and avoid holding your breath during any portion of a lift. The easiest technique for most to remember is to forcefully exhale during the hardest portion of the lift. For example, in the bench press, exhale while pushing the weight off your chest; in the leg press, exhale while pushing the weight forward. Again, it is tempting for many to hold their breath during the most difficult portion, but *do not do this!* Holding your breath while lifting can increase your blood pressure to dangerously high levels. It can also result in reduced blood flow to the heart or brain. If you feel dizzy at all during a resistance training test or a workout, you have probably held your breath too long and reduced blood flow to either of those important organs. If this happens, stop the workout and rest. Return only if you feel completely normal; reduce the amount of resistance during your next exercise or workout.

A one-repetition maximum (1RM) bench press and one-repetition maximum leg press have been used for years to determine strength. These tests are not recommended for some individuals who are older or have heart disease or severe hypertension because the test may result in temporary but significant elevation in blood pressure. A safer alternative would be to estimate single maximum lift with a submaximal test.

In order to perform the tests, make sure you are familiar with the proper technique and how to operate the equipment. You may even want to have a training partner or a fitness specialist (such as a personal trainer) help you. For the bench press test, begin with an easy warm-up, performing 10 to 12 repetitions using a relatively light weight. If you don't have previous experience with weight training, you'll need to select a starting weight by trial and error—if in doubt, err on the light side. Once you warm up, increase the resistance by about 20 to 30 pounds and perform a set of 7 to 10 repetitions. At the end of the set, it should be difficult, if not impossible, to complete another repetition. If you underestimated your first set, then increase again 10 to 20 pounds and repeat another 7 to 10 repetitions. To calculate your estimated 1RM use one of the following equations based on your level of weight-training experience (Braith et al. 1993).

Untrained

$$1RM = 1.554 \times 7\text{-}10 \text{ repetition weight (kg)} - 5.181$$

Trained

$$1RM = 1.172 \times 7\text{-}10 \text{ repetition weight (kg)} + 7.704$$

The same technique can be used to test your lower-body strength using a leg press. Record your best efforts for both exercises on your worksheet and then follow your specific program. See tables 3.2 and 3.3 to compare your numbers with normal 1RM values for your age and gender.

Table 3.2   Standard Values for 1RM Bench Press

Rank	Percentile	Age				
		20–29	30–39	40–49	50–59	Over 60
Men						
Superior	99	>1.63	>1.35	>1.20	>1.05	>.94
	95	1.63	1.35	1.20	1.05	.94
Excellent	90	1.48	1.24	1.10	.97	.89
	85	1.37	1.17	1.04	.93	.84
	80	1.32	1.12	1.00	.90	.82
Good	75	1.26	1.08	.96	.87	.79
	70	1.22	1.04	.93	.84	.77
	65	1.18	1.01	.90	.81	.74
	60	1.14	.98	.88	.79	.72
Fair	55	1.10	.96	.86	.77	.70
	50	1.06	.93	.84	.75	.68
	45	1.03	.90	.82	.73	.67
	40	.99	.88	.80	.71	.66

(continued)

Table 3.2   *(continued)*

Rank	Percentile	Age				
		20–29	30–39	40–49	50–59	Over 60
Men						
Poor	35	.96	.86	.78	.70	.65
	30	.93	.83	.76	.68	.63
	25	.90	.81	.74	.66	.60
	20	.88	.78	.72	.63	.57
Very poor	15	.84	.75	.69	.60	.56
	10	.80	.71	.65	.57	.53
	5	.72	.65	.59	.53	.49
	1	<.72	<.65	<.59	<.53	<.49
Women						
Superior	99	>1.01	>.82	>.77	>.68	>.72
	95	1.01	.82	.77	.68	.72
Excellent	90	.90	.76	.71	.61	.64
	85	.83	.72	.66	.57	.59
	80	.80	.70	.62	.55	.54
Good	75	.77	.65	.60	.53	.53
	70	.74	.63	.57	.52	.51
	65	.72	.62	.55	.50	.48
	60	.70	.60	.54	.48	.47
Fair	55	.68	.58	.53	.47	.46
	50	.65	.57	.52	.46	.45
	45	.63	.55	.51	.45	.44
	40	.59	.53	.50	.44	.43
Poor	35	.58	.52	.48	.43	.41
	30	.56	.51	.47	.42	.40
	25	.53	.49	.45	.41	.39
	20	.51	.47	.43	.39	.38
Very poor	15	.50	.45	.42	.38	.36
	10	.48	.42	.38	.37	.33
	5	.44	.39	.35	.31	.26
	1	<.44	<.39	<.35	<.31	<.26

Bench press weight ratio = weight pushed (pounds) divided by body weight (pounds)

Adapted, by permission, from The Cooper Institute, 2005, *Physical fitness specialist certification manual* (Dallas, TX: The Cooper Institute).

Table 3.3 Standard Values for 1RM Leg Press

Rank	Percentile	Age				
		20–29	30–39	40–49	50–59	Over 60
Men						
Superior	99	>2.40	>2.20	>2.02	>1.90	>1.80
	95	2.40	2.20	2.02	1.90	1.80
Excellent	90	2.27	2.07	1.92	1.80	1.73
	85	2.18	1.99	1.86	1.75	1.68
	80	2.13	1.93	1.82	1.71	1.62
Good	75	2.09	1.89	1.78	1.68	1.58
	70	2.05	1.85	1.74	1.64	1.56
	65	2.01	1.81	1.71	1.61	1.52
	60	1.97	1.77	1.68	1.58	1.49
Average	55	1.94	1.74	1.65	1.55	1.46
	50	1.91	1.71	1.62	1.52	1.43
	45	1.87	1.68	1.59	1.50	1.40
	40	1.83	1.65	1.57	1.46	1.38
Fair	35	1.78	1.62	1.54	1.42	1.34
	30	1.74	1.59	1.51	1.39	1.30
	25	1.68	1.56	1.48	1.36	1.27
	20	1.63	1.52	1.44	1.32	1.25
Poor	15	1.58	1.48	1.40	1.28	1.21
	10	1.51	1.43	1.35	1.22	1.16
	5	1.42	1.34	1.27	1.15	1.08
	1	<1.42	<1.34	<1.27	<1.15	<1.08

(continued)

Table 3.3   (continued)

Rank	Percentile	Age				
		20–29	30–39	40–49	50–59	Over 60
Women						
Superior	99	>1.98	>1.68	>1.57	>1.43	>1.43
	95	1.98	1.68	1.57	1.43	1.43
Excellent	90	1.82	1.61	1.48	1.37	1.32
	85	1.76	1.52	1.40	1.31	1.25
	80	1.68	1.47	1.37	1.25	1.18
Good	75	1.65	1.42	1.33	1.20	1.16
	70	1.58	1.39	1.29	1.17	1.13
	65	1.53	1.36	1.27	1.12	1.08
	60	1.50	1.33	1.23	1.10	1.04
Average	55	1.47	1.31	1.20	1.08	.99
	50	1.44	1.27	1.18	1.05	.99
	45	1.40	1.24	1.15	1.02	.97
	40	1.37	1.21	1.13	.99	.93
Fair	35	1.32	1.18	1.11	.97	.90
	30	1.27	1.15	1.08	.95	.90
	25	1.26	1.12	1.06	.92	.86
	20	1.22	1.09	1.02	.88	.85
Poor	15	1.18	1.05	.97	.84	.80
	10	1.14	1.00	.94	.78	.72
	5	.99	.96	.85	.72	.63
	1	<.99	<.96	<.85	<.72	<.63

Leg press weight ratio = weight pushed (pounds) divided by body weight (pounds)

Adapted, by permission, from The Cooper Institute, 2005, *Physical fitness specialist certification manual* (Dallas, TX: The Cooper Institue).

Testing Flexibility

For some, a measure of fitness is whether they can touch their toes; for others, fitness is whether they can *see* their toes! If you are in the former group, you would probably define yourself as flexible. Flexibility defines one's ability to move without stiffness or with what some refer to as "internal resistance." Our joints must always have a delicate balance of flexibility and stability: too stiff and movements are deliberate, painful, and slow; too flexible and our joints can dislocate.

For many years it has been believed that flexibility helps prevent injuries. It's unclear whether evidence truly supports this claim, but we do know that when certain areas, such as the hamstrings, calves, and lower back, are more flexible, chronic conditions like low-back pain and Achilles tendinitis are less of a problem. The upper-chest and shoulder area is frequently inflexible. In fact, almost all fatigue-related neck and upper-back pain—those tender "knots" that pop up beside your shoulder blades—are partially the result of inflexibility in the upper chest and fronts of the shoulders. Yet another commonly inflexible muscle group is the hip flexors. These powerful muscles are the largest and typically the strongest group in the body. We use the hip flexors most often to lift our thighs forward at the hip. Many people strengthen these muscles by doing sit-ups; however, in doing so they are unknowingly causing the hip flexors to be less flexible, which also contributes to chronic low-back pain.

Just as in the aerobic and resistance portions of your training program, you should establish a baseline level of flexibility before beginning your individualized flexibility program. In order to assess your flexibility we will use three tests: the sit-and-reach test, the hip flexor test, and the broomstick test. In order to get the most out of each test, have someone help you by measuring at the appropriate location for each test. You can compare your values to those in tables 3.4 and 3.5.

Sit-and-Reach Test

Begin by sitting on the floor, with your legs and knees straight in front of you, feet 8 to 10 inches apart. Some fitness clubs will have a small box to assist in this test. If you don't have this box available, place a yardstick on the floor with the starting point between your legs and the 15-inch mark even with your heels. Lean forward over your straight legs and reach as far as you can (see figure 3.2 on page 46). Have your spotter note how far you were able to reach as indicated by the measurements on the sit-and-reach box or the yardstick. After each reach, come back to the normal, nonreaching position, rest for a few seconds, and repeat the reach. Record your best distance of the three trials. Compare your score to the norms in table 3.4 and find your flexibility rating.

Table 3.4 Sit-and-Reach Ratings

Rank	Percentile	Age				
		20–29	30–39	40–49	50–59	Over 60
Men						
Superior	99	>23.0	>22.0	>21.3	>20.5	>20.0
	95	23.0	22.0	21.3	20.5	20.0
Excellent	90	21.8	21.0	20.0	19.0	19.0
	85	21.0	20.0	19.3	18.3	18.0
	80	20.5	19.5	18.5	17.5	17.3
Good	75	20.0	19.0	18.0	17.0	16.5
	70	19.5	18.5	17.5	16.5	15.5
	65	19.0	18.0	17.0	16.0	15.0
	60	18.5	17.5	16.3	15.5	14.5
Fair	55	18.0	17.0	16.0	15.0	14.0
	50	17.5	16.5	15.3	14.5	13.5
	45	17.0	16.0	15.0	14.0	13.0
	40	16.5	15.5	14.3	13.3	12.5
Poor	35	16.0	15.0	14.0	12.5	12.0
	30	15.5	14.5	13.3	12.0	11.3
	25	15.0	13.8	12.5	11.2	10.5
	20	14.4	13.0	12.0	10.5	10.0
Very poor	15	13.5	12.0	11.0	9.7	9.0
	10	12.3	11.0	10.0	8.5	8.0
	5	10.5	9.3	8.3	7.0	5.8
	1	<10.5	<9.3	<8.3	<7.0	<5.8

Rank	Percentile	Age				
		20–29	30–39	40–49	50–59	Over 60
Women						
Superior	99	>24.5	>24.0	>22.8	>23.0	>23.0
	95	24.5	24.0	22.8	23.0	23.0
Excellent	90	23.8	22.5	21.5	21.5	21.8
	85	23.0	22.0	21.3	21.0	19.5
	80	22.5	21.5	20.5	20.3	19.0
Good	75	22.0	21.0	20.0	20.0	18.0
	70	21.5	20.5	19.8	19.3	17.5
	65	21.0	20.3	19.1	19.0	17.5
	60	20.5	20.0	19.0	18.5	17.0
Fair	55	20.3	19.5	18.5	18.0	17.0
	50	20.0	19.0	18.0	17.9	16.4
	45	19.5	18.5	18.0	17.0	16.1
	40	19.3	18.3	17.3	16.8	15.5
Poor	35	19.0	17.8	17.0	16.0	15.2
	30	18.3	17.3	16.5	15.5	14.4
	25	17.8	16.8	16.0	15.3	13.6
	20	17.0	16.5	15.0	14.8	13.0
Very poor	15	16.4	15.5	14.0	14.0	11.5
	10	15.4	14.4	13.0	13.0	11.5
	5	14.1	12.0	10.5	12.3	9.2
	1	<14.1	<12.0	<10.5	<12.3	<9.2

Adapted, by permission, from The Cooper Institute, 2005, *Physical fitness specialist certification manual* (Dallas, TX: The Cooper Institue).

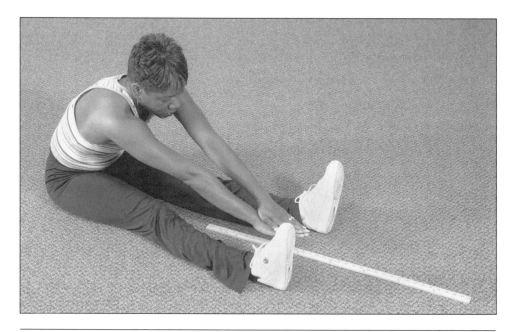

Figure 3.2   Proper technique for the sit-and-reach test.

Hip Flexor Test

This test is slightly more difficult to do than the sit-and-reach test, but it is easier to measure. Lie down on a firm bed or stable table with your buttocks at the edge and your knees bent and pulled toward your chest. Place your hands in the small of your back and try to keep them sandwiched between your back and the bed or table. One at a time, extend one leg forward as far as possible (see figure 3.3). Note what position the

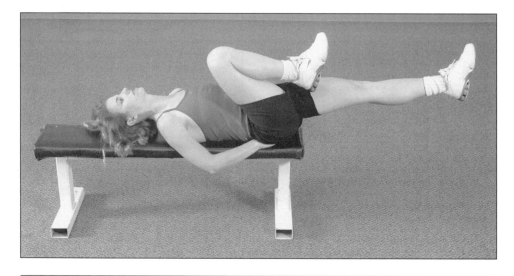

Figure 3.3   Proper technique for the hip flexor test.

straightened leg is in when you feel your lower back start to lift off your hand. Normally this occurs when your leg is in a straight line with your torso. If your leg extends farther and your knee descends lower than your torso before your lower back lifts off your hand, then you have above-average flexibility (and are in the minority). On the other hand, if the leg does not reach a straight line with your torso before your back lifts off your hand, then your flexibility is below average (welcome to the majority with the rest of us). There are no norm values for this test since there is no numerical measurement.

Broomstick Test

This test measures flexibility of your upper chest and shoulders. Find a broom or another lightweight, straight, thin object to hold in your hands during this test. Lie prone (facedown) on the floor. Extend your arms straight forward while holding the stick with your hands slightly wider than shoulder-width apart. Slowly raise the stick overhead (see figure 3.4). If you cannot raise your arms off the floor due to stiffness, this indicates below-average flexibility. If you are able to raise the stick slightly behind your head, this is average. Finally, if you can raise the stick well past your head, please stop, reduce your shoulders back into their respective sockets (I think I saw Mel Gibson do that in a movie once), and congratulate yourself for having above-average upper-body flexibility. If you want a more precise score, measure your arm length in inches as the distance from your acromial process (the bony point at the tip of your shoulder) to the tip of your longest finger. Once you have completed the arm raise test described above, subtract your vertical arm elevation score (the distance from the floor to your fingertips) from your arm length. Lower scores mean better flexibility. Compare your score to the values in table 3.5.

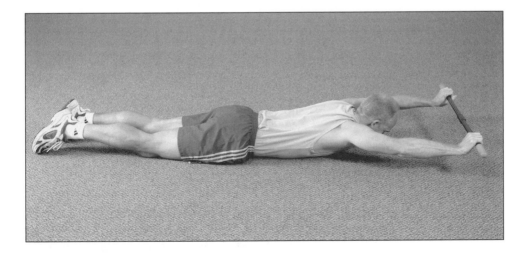

Figure 3.4 Proper technique for the broomstick test.

Table 3.5 Shoulder and Wrist Elevation Ratings

Rating	Men (scores in inches)	Women (scores in inches)
Excellent	<6	<5.5
Good	8.5–6.25	7.5–5.5
Average	11.5–8.5	10.5–7.5
Fair	12.5–11.5	12–10.5
Poor	>12.5	>12

Adapted, by permission, from W.D. McArdle, F.L. Katch and V.L. Katch, 1996, *Exercise physiology: Energy, nutrition and human performance,* 5th ed. (Baltimore, MD: Lippincott, Williams & Wilkins).

Measuring Body Composition

Your body composition is another important component in your quest to reduce your blood pressure by increasing your fitness. Body composition is a measurement of what percentage of your total body weight is fat. The average for middle-aged men is 17 to 22 percent, whereas women carry a little more fat and average 20 to 27 percent fat. Table 3.6 shows standard values for percentage of body fat; once you determine your body fat percentage, you can consult this table to see how healthy your percentage is.

There are several ways to measure percentage of body fat, but very few of them can be done accurately without someone else's help. The most scientifically accurate method uses the same technology that is used to measure bone density—dual energy X-ray absorptiometry (DEXA). DEXA scanning is a painless, easy, and accurate measurement, but very few centers use this technology at this time because of its high cost. If you have inexpensive access to DEXA scanning, take advantage of it.

Hydrostatic, or underwater, weighing is another accurate measurement that is less commonly used because of space and economic limitations of fitness centers. In this procedure, you are dressed in a swimsuit and submerged completely under water. If being under water for about 30 seconds is a problem for you—and it is for many—this is not the method for you. Again, if you have inexpensive access to this test, take advantage of it, as this is another accurate means of measuring percentage of body fat.

Skinfold measurements are perhaps the most accurate of the more commonly used techniques for measuring body fat. Using specialized calipers, a trained technician will measure skinfold thickness at three to eight predetermined sites on the body. These measurements, along with your age and body weight, are then used in an equation to predict your

Table 3.6 Standard Values for Percentage of Body Fat

Rating	Age				
	20–29	30–39	40–49	50–59	Over 60
Men					
Excellent	<10	<11	<13	<14	<15
Good	11–13	12–14	14–16	15–17	16–18
Average	14–20	15–21	17–23	18–24	19–25
Fair	21–23	22–24	24–26	25–27	26–28
Poor	>24	>25	>27	>28	>29
Women					
Excellent	<15	<16	<17	<18	<19
Good	16–19	17–20	18–21	19–22	20–23
Average	20–28	21–29	22–30	23–31	24–32
Fair	29–31	30–32	31–33	32–34	33–35
Poor	>32	>33	>34	>35	>36

Reprinted, by permission, from A.S. Jackson, M.L. Pollock and A. Ward, 1980, "Generalized equations for predicting body density of women," *Med Sci Sports Exerc* 12(3): 175-182; reprinted, by permission, from A.S. Jackson and M.L. Pollock, 1978, "Generalized equations for predicting body density of men," *Br J Nutr* 40(3): 497-504.

percentage of body fat. In the hands of a well-trained technician, skinfold measurements can be nearly as accurate as hydrostatic weighing. Skinfold measurements are ideal because the cost is low and the space required is minimal.

Another common but less accurate method of measuring percentage of body fat is to use commercially available impedance devices. Using the basic principles of electricity, your impedance, or resistance to electrical flow, is estimated and then correlated to the amount of body fat. Not as accurate as the other methods, impedance measurements are very much affected by hydration: if you are underhydrated, your body fat measurement can be off by as much as 6 percent. Several companies use this technology in home bathroom scales and for health screenings as a way to individually monitor percentage of body fat. Again, the technology is not that accurate, and results should be taken with a grain of salt. Having a home body impedance measuring device is not essential in your quest, so spend the money more wisely on something else.

Currently, the accepted way to grade the level of overweight is to measure the *body mass index (BMI)*. Physicians, therapists, and insurance companies use BMI as a way to categorize your body as underweight, overweight, obese, or just right. These classifications, along with waist size as discussed in a few paragraphs, correspond to level of risk for diabetes, high blood pressure, and heart disease (see table 3.7). The BMI number is based on your height in proportion to your weight using the following calculation (see also the tables in the appendix for BMI values, pages 171-173):

$$BMI = [\text{weight in pounds} \div (\text{height in inches} \times \text{height in inches})] \times 703$$

For example, for a person weighing 150 pounds who is 5 feet, 9 inches tall, the calculation would be as follows:

$$[150 \div (69 \times 69)] \times 703 = 22$$

It is important to apply this number with caution. For example, well over half of the players in the NFL would be classified as obese based on their BMIs, even the players with less than 10 percent body fat. Clearly, having less body fat is preferable to having a lower BMI. On the other end, your weight may well be in proportion to your height, giving you an ideal, or even low, BMI (this does not happen too often, but it does occasionally), but your body fat may be over 30 percent because you have never exercised and have very little muscle mass. These are the two extremes, and most of us do fall within the acceptable categories. Current medical research most often uses BMI to classify the body composition of research

Table 3.7 Risk of Associated Disease According to BMI and Waist Size

BMI	Weight classification	Waist less than or equal to 40 inches (men) or 35 inches (women)	Waist greater than 40 inches (men) or 35 inches (women)
18.5 or less	Underweight	--	N/A
18.5–24.9	Normal	--	N/A
25.0–29.9	Overweight	Increased	High
30.0–34.9	Obese	High	Very high
35.0–39.9	Obese	Very high	Very high
40 or greater	Extremely obese	Extremely high	Extremely high

Reprinted, by permission, from WHO (World Health Organization), 1997, "Obesity: Preventing and Managing the Global Epidemic of Obesity."

▷ Assessment Score Sheet

Record your score for the applicable tests in the blanks below. Use this form each time you take the assessments, and then compare scores to track your improvement.

AEROBIC CAPACITY TESTS

Rockport 1-Mile Walk Test

Weight _____ pounds

Age _____ years

Walk time ___:___ minutes:seconds

HR _____ beats per minute

132.853 − (0.0769 × weight [lb]) − (0.3877 × age [yr]) + (6.315 × 0 [females] or 1 [males]) − (3.2649 × time [min]) − (0.1565 × HR) = _____ ($\dot{V}O_2$max)

Comments_____

Stationary Cycle Test

Revolutions per minute _____

Heart rate 1 _____ beats per minute

Heart rate 2 _____ beats per minute

$\dot{V}O_2$max _____

Comments_____

MUSCULAR STRENGTH TESTS

1RM Bench Press

7-10 repetition weight _____ pounds

Untrained: 1.554 × 7-10 repetition weight (kg) − 5.181 = _____ (1RM)

Trained: 1.172 × 7-10 repetition weight (kg) + 7.704 = _____ (1RM)

Comments_____

1RM Leg Press

7-10 repetition weight _____ pounds

Untrained: 1.554 × 7-10 repetition weight (kg) − 5.181 = _____ (1RM)

Trained: 1.172 × 7-10 repetition weight (kg) + 7.704 = _____ (1RM)

Comments_____

FLEXIBILITY TESTS

Sit-and-Reach Test

Best score (of three tries) _____ inches

Comments_____

(continued)

Hip Flexor Test

Position of leg at end of test _____

Comments_____

Broomstick Test

Vertical arm elevation (distance between floor and fingertips) _____ inches

Arm length _____ inches

Score (arm length – arm elevation) _____

Comments_____

BODY COMPOSITION TESTS

Percentage of Body Fat

Method of measurement _____

Percent body fat _____

Body Mass Index

Weight _____ pounds

Height _____ inches

[weight in pounds ÷ (height in inches × height in inches)] × 703 = _____
  (BMI)

Comments_____

From *Action Plan for High Blood Pressure* by Jon G. Divine, 2006, Champaign, IL: Human Kinetics.

subjects and to establish the predicted risk of other health conditions, such as hypertension, with being overweight or obese. Almost certainly, if you reduce your BMI through a smart program of exercise and healthy eating, your blood pressure and the risks associated with elevated blood pressure will be lower.

Waist circumference is another predictor of percentage of body fat. A decade ago, researchers looked at the waist-to-hip measurements and generally categorized individuals by their shape: either apple shaped (tending to store fat in the middle of the body) or pear shaped (tending to store fat in the thighs and buttocks). Those who were apple shaped had a higher amount of intra-abdominal fat storage and were at higher risk of type 2 (also known as adult-onset) diabetes, high blood pressure, and heart disease compared to those who were pear shaped (see table 3.7).

Summary

The tasks we have accomplished in this chapter are significant in the process of improving your blood pressure by improving your strength, flexibility, body weight, and overall fitness. These tests will be some of the yardsticks with which you can measure your success in taking control of your blood pressure. More important, these results will allow you to individualize your exercise prescription. The self-test results you record now on your assessment worksheet will be both interesting and rewarding to look back on in the next few months as you progress through your exercise program. The other yardstick will be the most challenging, yet sounds so easy: follow the program. That's it: Just follow the daily routine you have set ahead of yourself, and you will be on your way toward active blood pressure control.

ACTION PLAN:
ASSESSING YOUR FITNESS LEVEL

☐ Schedule your annual physical exam when appropriate to discuss with your doctor your current health status and your exercise and diet plans.

☐ Choose from the following aerobic capacity tests:

- Rockport 1-Mile Walk Test
- Stationary Cycle Tests

☐ Perform the one-repetition maximum bench press and leg press tests to assess your strength.

☐ Select a test to evaluate your flexibility from the following choices:

- Sit-and-reach test
- Hip flexor test
- Broomstick test

☐ Compare your aerobic, strength, and flexibility test scores to established norms to determine your fitness level in these areas.

☐ Determine the most convenient and accurate way to have your body composition measured.

☐ Use the information obtained in this chapter as a baseline for customizing the details of your exercise program.

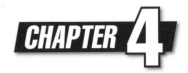

CHAPTER 4

REGULATING PRESSURE THROUGH AEROBIC ACTIVITY

Simply stated, aerobic means "with oxygen." We are aerobic beings. Everything we do, every movement, every thought, every heartbeat, every millimeter of digestive tract movement requires the delivery of oxygen to working cells. We are so dependent on oxygen that without it for more than a few minutes, our cells will die. Many cells have the capability to become more efficient with the delivered oxygen by adapting to greater workloads. The skeletal muscle is the classic example. Just as a muscle gradually becomes bigger as it lifts more weight over time, the internal aerobic machinery of the muscle also grows and becomes more efficient.

Muscles (and many other cell types) also have a reserve that allows them to function without oxygen, or *anaerobically,* for a few minutes. The classic example of this is the sprinter who runs 100 meters in 10 seconds. There is simply not enough time to deliver the necessary oxygen to the working muscle in less than 10 seconds, and the body does not have the capacity to breathe in and use the oxygen it would take to run 100 meters in 10 seconds. What we do have is the capability to do this and many other quick, sudden, strenuous activities without oxygen. But we have limited ability to do this, so we can sustain these activities only for up to 2 or 3 minutes before we are completely fatigued and out of breath. Most of our strenuous short occupation tasks fall into this anaerobic activity range. Although regular anaerobic activity is good, especially if you are a sprinter or a weightlifter, it offers few benefits (if any) for regulating your blood pressure. That is why this chapter focuses on aerobic exercise, which is proven to help maintain healthy blood pressure.

How Aerobic Exercise Lowers Blood Pressure

In chapter 2 we discussed how regular aerobic exercise specifically affects blood pressure. During an aerobic workout, heart rate and blood pressure increase to meet the demands for increased oxygen at the level of the working muscles. The exercising pressure rises due to the increase in heart rate and in stroke volume, or amount of blood pumped per beat. The force of each heart contraction also increases. Blood flow to the active muscles is increased as blood vessels to active body tissues widen and blood vessels to inactive or nonessential body tissues become narrower. Resistance to blood flow generally decreases during exercise. An individual's maximum oxygen utilization capacity, or $\dot{V}O_2max$, increases as he or she gets more fit.

Resting blood pressure is improved through regular aerobic exercise because the body adapts to performing more strenuous activities or higher workloads by growing more blood vessels to supply the blood and oxygen demands of the working muscles. Plasma volume increases, which allows more blood to be returned to the heart, which in turn allows it to pump a higher volume of blood with each stroke. Cardiac output then increases at rest and with exercise. The total peripheral resistance decreases to allow more efficient delivery of oxygenated blood to working muscles.

The decrease in blood flow resistance occurring during a workout carries over into the postexercise period, resulting in lower systolic and diastolic blood pressure up to 22 hours after a workout. Exercising regularly enables you to have more time with the lower pressure.

In order to achieve the benefits of exercise, you must commit time to regular exercise and maintain it as part of your lifestyle. The stored energy in the form of fat is used like a big pile of coal (or an environmentally friendly form of fuel) to fuel all your extra activity, both at rest and with activity. With consistent exercise, you will become a more efficient mover and exerciser and your time commitment will be rewarded. But these changes don't occur overnight; it takes time to achieve these benefits of regular aerobic exercise. Most of these training effects take at least two and sometimes up to six weeks to achieve.

Do not forget about the calorie burning that comes with exercise and activity. Researchers estimate that if you burn an extra 2,000 calories per week, your life expectancy is about seven years longer than that of those who do not burn the extra calories. And the chances of those extra years being quality years (including your sex life) are also much greater if you are more active earlier in life. The weight loss that comes through burning extra calories is another positive factor for blood pressure reduction.

Determining Aerobic Exercise Dosage

If regular exercise is a drug, then the aerobic type is the most powerful one when it comes to affecting blood pressure. To expand the medication metaphor, the type of exercise is just as important in lowering blood pressure as the type of medicine is for a condition, according to the principle of specificity discussed in chapter 2. Exercise must be "taken" on a regular basis, preferably daily. There is a dose-related response to exercise on several of the body's systems—most important, the cardiovascular system. The exercise intensity combined with the total amount of exercise done in one session equals the "dosage" of daily exercise. We'll discuss in the following sections the best dosage—frequency, time, and intensity—for affecting blood pressure.

Frequency and Time

Research shows that just as medicine has an ideal or most effective dose, so too does exercise. The more time you put in, the more beneficial the adapted response, especially when it comes to lowering blood pressure. The minimum threshold to achieve this dose-related response of exercise on blood pressure is generally accepted to be about 30 minutes per day. The blood pressure response improves with more exercise up to about 60 minutes. After 60 minutes, there is less response. Recent research has shown that at least three bouts of 10 minutes of exercise during the day has the same benefit as one 30-minute session. This 30 to 60 minutes would be considered the best duration for positive blood pressure effects.

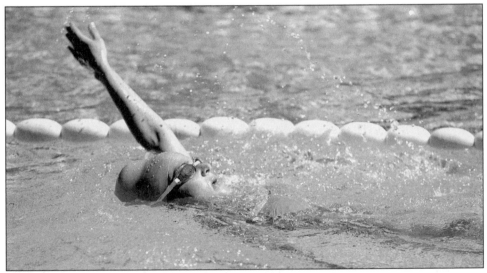

© Photodisc

Blood pressure is most positively affected with 30 to 60 minutes of aerobic exercise, such as swimming, three to five days of the week.

Remember that there is a time period of about one day following 30 to 60 minutes of exercise in which blood pressure is lower than before the exercise, and after that the blood pressure returns to normal. So in order to develop the adaptive blood pressure response that occurs with regular exercise, the 30 minutes of exercise must be repeated regularly. Three times weekly should be the minimum goal, and daily is ideal. Put into a weekly time perspective, to achieve ideal blood pressure control from exercise would take about two and a half to seven hours per week.

Intensity

The other half of your exercise dosage is intensity. To many, the message that you don't need to run or jog to achieve fitness is getting through. Examples of this can be seen by the increasing numbers who meet their fitness needs by simply walking continuously for 20 to 60 minutes. For most, a walk at 3 or 4 miles per hour represents 40 to 60 percent of maximum functional capacity ($\dot{V}O_2$max). And researchers tell us that in order for exercise to benefit our blood pressure, exercise intensity should be about 40 to 60 percent of our maximum functional capacity. It doesn't take much. Exercising beyond 70 to 80 percent of maximum has benefits on the system but does not add any additional benefit to blood pressure control. So you don't really need to sprint around the block; walking will do just fine.

Measuring Intensity With Metabolic Equivalents

The difficulty for many is in determining how much activity represents the ideal 40 to 60 percent exercise intensity range. To simplify this, the energy required to do many activities has been measured and normalized into units called METs (metabolic equivalents). Basically, this is an approximate assignment of the caloric value of an activity. One MET is the amount of oxygen you use at rest. The higher the MET, the higher the intensity. In order to determine the ideal training intensity, you need to have an idea of your functional capacity value ($\dot{V}O_2$max). This is obtained from your performance on any of the aerobic capacity tests discussed in chapter 3. To determine your max METs, simply divide your $\dot{V}O_2$max number by 3.5. For example, if your initial $\dot{V}O_2$max is estimated at 25 ml/kg/min, this makes your max METs about 7.1 METs. The level of intensity you will be able to sustain is somewhere between 40 and 60 percent of your max METs.

Beginners, take your estimated or measured maximum functional capacity value and multiply it by 40 percent. From here, you can go to table 4.1 and find activities that closely approximate your range. If your preferred activity is not included in this table, check out the following Web site, which contains an extensive listing of activities' MET levels: www.cdc.gov/nccdphp/dnpa/physical/pdf/PA_Intensity_table_2_1.pdf.

Table 4.1 Metabolic Equivalents of Selected Activities

Activity	METs used
Bicycling outdoors, <10.0 mph, leisure riding	4.0
Bicycling outdoors, 10.0–11.9 mph	6.0
Bicycling outdoors, 12.0–13.9 mph	8.0
Bicycling outdoors, 14.0–15.9 mph	10.0
Biking, stationary, 50 watts, very light effort	3.0
Biking, stationary, 100 watts, light effort	5.5
Biking, stationary, 150 watts, moderate effort	7.0
Biking, stationary, 200 watts, vigorous effort	10.5
Running, 5 mph	8.0
Running, 6 mph	10.0
Running, 7 mph	11.5
Running, 8 mph	13.5
Swimming laps, freestyle, moderate to light effort	8.0
Swimming laps, sidestroke	8.0
Swimming laps, backstroke	8.0
Swimming laps, breaststroke	10.0
Swimming laps, butterfly	11.0
Walking, 2.0 mph	2.5
Walking, 2.5 mph	3.0
Walking, 3.0 mph	3.5
Walking, 3.5 mph	4.0
Walking, 4.5 mph	4.5

Adapted, by permission, from American College of Sports Medicine (ACSM), 2001, *ACSM's resource manual for guidelines for exercise testing and prescription,* 4th ed. (Baltimore, MD: Lippincott, Williams & Wilkins), 674-681.

Monitoring Intensity With Heart Rate Measurements

Another way to monitor your intensity is to measure your exercising heart rate. The ideal training or target heart rate (THR) range is 50 to 85 percent of maximum, and there is no added benefit to blood pressure by exercising so intensely that your heart rate is above 85 percent of maximum. A commonly used estimate of maximum heart rate (HRmax) is to subtract your age from 220. For example, the maximum heart rate for a 40-year-old is 180 beats per minute. However, if you had a stress test in which you achieved a maximum heart rate, you would use the maximum *achieved* heart rate.

What should your heart rate be for a given exercise intensity? Subtract your resting heart rate (RHR) from your maximum heart rate. Let's define your resting heart rate as the rate taken after you have sat upright quietly for 10 minutes. The difference between your maximum heart rate and resting heart rate is multiplied by the percentage of desired exercise intensity. To that value, your resting heart rate is added back, and this new value is your training heart rate. In other words, you would use this equation:

$$\text{HRmax} - \text{RHR} \times \text{intensity (percent)} + \text{RHR} = \text{THR}$$

For example, a 50-year-old with a maximum heart rate of 170 and a resting heart rate of 60 who wants to see what his heart rate should be when exercising at 50 percent of maximum functional capacity would use the following equation:

$$170 - 60 = 110$$
$$110 \times .5 \text{ (50 percent)} = 55$$
$$55 + 60 = 115 \text{ beats per minute (target heart rate)}$$

If this 50-year-old had a very good maximal functional capacity of 10 METs, 50 percent would be 5 METs. Examples of 5-MET activities include recreationally shooting a basketball (not playing a game of basketball), square dancing, and walking on a treadmill at 4 MPH flat or 3.5 MPH with a 5 percent grade. This 50-year-old's heart rate should then be about 115 plus or minus about 5 beats per minute. If this 50-year-old could do these activities for at least 30 to 60 minutes about three to seven times in one week, he could expect to see changes in condition, body weight, and blood pressure in about four to six weeks.

How do you make sure you're hitting your calculated target heart rate during exercise? During exercise your best speedometer is your heart rate. It is your most accurate reflection as to how hard or easy a workout or workload has become. It takes about 5 to 10 minutes for heart rate to plateau for a constant workload. So if, for example, you have completed your warm-up and have begun the aerobic portion of your workout and have stayed fairly consistent in your pace or workload, check your heart rate at 10 minutes. If the heart rate is lower than your target range you can speed up, or increase the workload, and check again in 10 minutes. If, on the other hand, the heart rate is too high, slow down your pace or workload and check again in 10 minutes. Remember, another easy guideline to indicate whether you are working too hard is that the intensity of the workout should be such that you can carry on a normal conversation while exercising without becoming more short of breath.

Measuring Intensity by How You Feel

With practice, the Borg rating of perceived exertion scale can be the easiest method for determining how hard you are working during your workout. After your level of exercise intensity has plateaued during a workout, usually after about 10 minutes at a constant intensity, simply rate how hard you feel you are working, given the verbal descriptions listed in figure 4.1. This self-description of the current workload is assigned a number from 6 to 20. Oddly enough, by adding a 0 to the exertion number (6 to 20) you will have a well-correlated estimate of your current heart rate. This is an important means of determining exertion levels for those who are taking medications for blood pressure or heart rate control, such as beta-blockers, because the medication keeps the exercising heart rate lower. In other words, despite working hard and feeling like you are working hard, the medication keeps your exercising heart rate at a lower rate. Regardless of whether you are taking rate-control medication, as you become more fit your exertion level will decrease for the same exercise program. In order to maintain progress toward increased fitness, the level of work, and thus the level of exertion, will need to increase (more on this in a later section).

6	No exertion at all
7	
8	Extremely light
9	Very light
10	
11	Light
12	
13	Somewhat hard
14	
15	Hard (heavy)
16	
17	Very hard
18	
19	Extremely hard
20	Maximal exertion

Borg RPE scale
© Gunnar Borg, 1970, 1985, 1994, 1998

Figure 4.1   Borg's rating of perceived exertion scale.

G. Borg, 1998, *Borg's perceived exertion and pain scales* (Champaign, IL: Human Kinetics), 47.

Progression

As we discussed in chapter 2, you need to gradually increase your workload as your training progresses. Remember, your body adapts to the added workload, so the amount of exercise that represents 40 percent of your maximal capacity at the beginning of your program may represent only 36 percent in six weeks. This does not indicate much of a change, probably an increase of about a 0.5 MPH faster walking pace. Fortunately, you don't need to add time to continue the adaptive process and improved benefits for blood pressure. Still, many do increase their workout times because they gradually begin to enjoy the training and find a way to prioritize additional daily training time. Again, don't forget that the amount of calories burned per workout continues to increase with the amount of time spent exercising. Adding an extra 20 minutes to a workout usually results in an increased calorie burn of about 150 calories. That's about 5 to 10 pounds extra lost per year, which can equate to approximately a 4- to 8-mmHg decrease in blood pressure. That might be enough for some to be able to cease the medication they thought they would take for the rest of their days.

Aerobic Exercise Programs

Because regular exercise is an essential ingredient in the medical management of hypertension, everyone with chronic hypertension should adopt some principles and techniques that athletes use. Athletes train daily at the appropriate intensity level, generally for about one or two hours per workout. They follow appropriate, well-planned training programs, and most are under the guidance of a coach. Too much exercise puts too much stress on the system, causing the body to break down instead of improving. Athletes do their best not to undertrain or overtrain. Adequate rest between workouts is just as important as the workout itself, in order to completely recover and train another day. Equally important is the athlete's diet and "refueling" between workouts. Taking into account all of these factors, we provide some programs here for walking, running, cycling, and swimming. Use these sample programs as they are or as a springboard for customizing your own program.

Walking

Walking is one of the most popular forms of aerobic exercise, in part because of its convenience. All you need are good supportive shoes and a place to walk. Walking can be done outside on a walking path or in your neighborhood, or inside on a treadmill or indoor track. People often find that walking with a friend increases the enjoyment of it.

The sample programs we provide in table 4.2 encompass three levels—low, medium, and high. Your $\dot{V}O_2$max score will tell you your fitness level (see page 35) and thus which program best matches your abilities.

Table 4.2 Sample Walking Program

Week	Frequency (times per week)	Distance (miles)	Speed (minutes-per-mile pace)	Time (minutes)
Low level				
1	3	0.75	20	15
2	3	1	20	20
3	3	1.25	20	25
4	4	1.25	20	25
5	4	1.5	20	30
6	4	1.75	20	35
7	5	1.75	20	35
8	5	2	20	40
9	5	2.25	20	45
10	5	2.25	20	45
Medium level				
1	3	1	20	20
2	3	1.25	20	25
3	3	1.5	20	30
4	4	1.5	20	30
5	4	1.75	20	35
6	4	2	17.5	35
7	5	2	17.5	35
8	5	2.25	17.5	40
9	5	2.5	17.5	45
10	5	2.5	17.5	45
High level				
1	3	1.25	17.5	20
2	3	1.5	17.5	25
3	3	1.75	17.5	30
4	4	1.75	17.5	30
5	4	2	15	30
6	4	2.25	15	35
7	5	2.25	15	35
8	5	2.5	15	40
9	5	2.75	15	43
10	5	3	15	45

Running

If you have completed the 30-week walking program, or are in condition and up for an additional challenge, then running may be for you. Runners are some of the most dedicated exercisers. Whether in sun, rain, wind, or snow, runners are most likely to exercise regularly, if not daily, than any other group of athletes. Running is not fast walking. The energy requirement is twice that of walking and results in two to eight times the force of body weight per stride. That is a lot of work. However, if you are up for it, running is the most efficient exercise method for burning calories. Blood pressure elevation is rarely an issue for those who run this far, usually because they weigh less, don't smoke, and burn about 3,500 to 5,000 calories per week! Runners who run 15 to 35 miles per week have an extremely low risk of heart disease.

The chances of overuse injury are, however, greater in runners than walkers and increase in proportion to the amount of mileage per week. Heavier runners tend to be injured more often than lighter runners. Other factors that may influence injury rate in runners include poor lower-body and hip strength, poor flexibility, foot pronation, and excessively flat or high-arched feet. By far, the factor having the most influence on injury is the amount of training volume increase per week. As volume increases beyond 10 percent per week, the rate of injury goes up. A 50 percent increase in weekly volume is almost guaranteed to result in injury within four weeks! So to better assure training success, the smart runner will not exceed the 10 percent rule.

Beginning runners, graduates of the walking program, or persons with fitness levels lower than average for their age (according to table 3.1) should begin with the low-level program in table 4.3. Walking program graduates with average to above-average fitness can begin with the medium-level program. Experienced runners, those who complete the low- or medium-level programs who want to run faster, and individuals with above-average levels of fitness can tackle the high-level program.

Cycling

If you're like me, the only time you run is from angry animals and the police. Just kidding—some of my best friends and family are law enforcement professionals. Seriously, to some, the relatively slow change of scenery associated with running can be boring. Others may be on the larger side and don't do well with the pounding of their lower extremities against the ground. Some have already pounded their lower extremities into an arthritic state and can't run without discomfort or pain. If this describes you, then cycling can be the best thing going. It takes at least a $100 investment in a bike worth riding—above that, the amount spent on accessorizing is up to you. Cycling certainly is for those who prefer the outdoors, so those who only ride need to be prepared for the changes in weather.

Table 4.3 Sample Running Program

Week	Jog/walk	Miles	Time (minutes)	Frequency (times per week)	Estimated calories burned per workout	Calories burned per week
Low level: 12-minute-mile pace						
1	Jog 1/2 mile, walk 1/2 mile, jog 1/2 mile, walk 1/2 mile, jog 1/2 mile	2.5	20–30	3	202	606
2	Jog 3/4 mile, walk 1/2 mile, jog 3/4 mile, walk 1/2 mile	2.5	25–35	3	252.5	757.5
3	Jog 1 mile, walk 1/2 mile, jog 1 mile	2.5	30–35	3	303	909
4	Jog 1 mile, walk 1/2 mile, jog 1 mile	2.5	30–35	4	303	1,212
5	Jog 1 1/4 miles, walk 1/2 mile, jog 1 1/4 miles	3	35–40	4	323.2	1,292.8
6	Jog 1 1/2 miles, walk 1/2 mile, jog 1 1/2 miles	3.5	40–45	4	353.5	1,414
7	Jog 1 1/2 miles, walk 1/2 mile, jog 1 1/2 miles	3.5	40–45	5	404	2,020
8	Jog 2 miles	2	20–30	5	242.4	1,212
Total weight lost: 2.69 pounds						
Medium level: 10-minute-mile pace						
1	Jog 1/2 mile, walk 1/2 mile, jog 1/2 mile, walk 1/2 mile, jog 1/2 mile	2.5	20–30	3	202.07	606.21
2	Jog 3/4 mile, walk 1/2 mile, jog 3/4 mile, walk 1/2 mile	2.5	20–30	3	261.51	784.53
3	Jog 1 mile, walk 1/2 mile, jog 1 mile	2.5	30	3	297.17	891.51
4	Jog 1 mile, walk 1/2 mile, jog 1 mile	2.5	30	4	297.17	1,188.68
5	Jog 1 1/4 miles, walk 1/2 mile, jog 1 1/4 miles	3	35–40	4	320.94	1,283.76
6	Jog 1 1/2 miles, walk 1/2 mile, jog 1 1/2 miles	3.5	35–40	4	416.03	1,664.12
7	Jog 1 1/2 miles, walk 1/2 mile, jog 1 1/2 miles	3.5	35–40	5	416.03	2,080.15
8	Jog 2 miles	2	20	5	237.73	1,188.65
Total weight lost: 2.77 pounds						

(continued)

Table 4.3 *(continued)*

Week	Jog/walk	Miles	Time (minutes)	Frequency (times per week)	Estimated calories burned per workout	Calories burned per week
High level: <8-minute-mile pace						
1	Jog 1 mile, walk 1/2 mile, jog 1 mile	2.5	20–30	3	291.33	873.99
2	Jog 1 mile, walk 1/2 mile, jog 1 mile	2.5	20–30	3	291.33	873.99
3	Jog 1 1/4 miles, walk 1/2 mile, jog 1 1/4 miles	3	30–35	3	349.6	1,048.8
4	Jog 1 1/2 miles, walk 1/2 mile, jog 1 1/2 miles	3.5	30–35	4	349.6	1,398.4
5	Jog 1 1/2 miles, walk 1/2 mile, jog 1 1/2 miles	3.5	30–35	4	422.43	1,689.72
6	Jog 2 miles	2	15–20	4	291.33	1,165.32
7	Jog 2 miles, walk 1/2 mile, jog 1 mile	3.5	30–35	5	422.43	2,112.15
8	Jog 2 1/2 miles, walk 1/2 mile, jog 1 mile	4	35–40	5	466.13	2,330.65
9	Jog 4 miles	4	30–40	5	466.13	2,330.65
Total weight lost: 3.95 pounds						

When compared to running, the body stays cooler riding in the heat, but riding in the cold can be a much greater challenge. There is a relative increase in the wind-chill factor by cutting through the cold air at 10 to 20 MPH. Speaking of wind resistance, the bigger your surface area—and we all know who we are—there is an increased cooling effect at the cost of an increase in the work needed to pedal against the wind. Despite these apparent hardships, there is no better way to explore an area either on the road or off.

Cyclists need to be most conscious of their safety when sharing the road with cars. Those riding bikes need to follow the same traffic rules as drivers: stay to the right, stop at all stop signs and red lights, pass on the left, and of course obey the speed limit! When riding at night or before sunrise, use a light and wear reflective clothing. A good safety rule of thumb for cyclists is to *always be seen.* Cyclists need to be more observant and anticipate what their auto-driving brethren are going to do. This is especially important in high-traffic areas and all intersections.

Much like the importance of correct running shoe fit, a well-fitted bike is essential for those who plan to cycle regularly. Expert bike fitting can be found at most bike shops and should be ensured before any bike purchase. The frame crossbar should be about 1 inch lower than your crotch when straddling the crossbar, out of the seat. The seat height should be adjusted so the knee has only a slight bend present in pull extension (when the pedal is in the lowest position). The handlebars should be adjusted to comfort. Novice riders will prefer a more upright seated position with very little forward lean or reach. Experienced riders prefer a more aerodynamic position bent over the bars with the shoulders forward. In addition to proper fit, regularly inspecting the bike's moving parts and stopping parts (brakes!) will assure you a safe ride and return.

If you want to add cycling to your workout plan, select your program (see table 4.4) based on your fitness assessment results. It is OK to use the results of a walking or running test to select where to begin your cycling program. If you find that your program becomes more of a cycling program, you may want to do subsequent assessments on a stationary bike.

If you love cycling and want to take your skill to the next level, I recommend *Serious Cycling, Second Edition,* by Edmund Burke (2002). This book contains a wealth of information on cycling technique, biomechanics, and training. Some top cycling coaches have benefited from Dr. Burke's years of research and knowledge about the science of cycling. If getting your own cycling coach is not in the budget for this year, strongly consider reading this book.

Table 4.4 Sample Cycling Program

Week	Miles	Time (minutes)	Frequency (times per week)	Estimated calories burned per workout	Calories burned per week
Low level: 60–80 RPM; <12 MPH; 55–75 watts; 4–5.5 cal/min					
1	3–4	20–30	3	123.96	371.88
2	3–4	25–35	3	148.75	446.25
3	5–6	30–35	3	173.54	520.62
4	5–6	30–35	4	173.54	694.16
5	7–8	35–40	4	183.46	733.84
6	7–8	40–45	4	208.25	833
7	7–8	40–45	5	208.25	1,041.25
8	8–10	45–60	5	252.88	1,264.4
Total weight lost: 1.69 pounds					

(continued)

Table 4.4   *(continued)*

Week	Miles	Time (minutes)	Frequency (times per week)	Estimated calories burned per workout	Calories burned per week
Medium level: 70–90 RPM; 12–16 MPH; 85–140 watts; 6–9 cal/min					
1	4.5–7	20–30	3	185	555
2	4.5–7	25–30	3	199.8	599.4
3	7	30	3	222	666
4	7–8	30–35	4	259	1,036
5	8–10.5	35–40	4	273.8	1,095.2
6	8–10.5	35–40	4	273.8	1,095.2
7	8–10.5	35–40	5	296	1,480
8	10–12	40–45	5	333	1,665
Total weight lost: 2.34 pounds					
High level: 80–100+ RPM; 16 MPH; 100–200 watts; 7–12.5 cal/min					
1	8–10	20–30	3	245	735
2	8–10	20–30	3	264.6	793.8
3	8–10	30–35	3	313.6	940.8
4	8–10	30–35	4	343	1,372
5	8–10	35–40	4	392	1,568
6	10–20	45–60	4	441	1,764
7	10–20	45–60	5	441	2,205
8	10–20	50–60	5	490	2,450
9	10–20	50–60	5	588	2,940
Total weight lost: 4.22 pounds					

Swimming

Swimmers are another group of dedicated athletes. People who swim have a natural comfort in the water that allows them to perform consistently and follow a regular routine that allows them to stay in top shape. They like, if not love, the water. They have no fear of water, can float very well, and can comfortably hold their breath under water without panic for 30 to 60 seconds. Swimmers place little force on their lower extremities. Their shoulders, however, can take a beating if their technique is less than perfect. Certainly, swimming is not for everyone. Adults who did not learn to swim as children have difficulty developing the skills required to swim. Once the fear factor is tamed, they seem to be able to learn the skills. If you want to learn to swim, take lessons before you commit yourself to adding swimming to your fitness routine.

No special equipment, besides a large body of clean water, is needed. Competitive swimmers can swim up to 10,000 to 12,000 meters per workout. Novices do not need or want to swim that far, or very fast. A good swimming workout distance of about 1,000 to 2,000 meters is very good for most. Swimming speed affects exercising heart rate: an important note is that exercising heart rate is about 5 to 10 percent lower while horizontal in the pool than during upright walking, running, or cycling exercise. Therefore, for about the same amount of exercise intensity as exercise on dry land, your heart rate will be lower in the pool. The exception to this would be those who swim outside with waves or a current; these factors increase exercise heart rate. If you are a beginner, skip the waves and swim in a pool. The added effects of current and waves are too unpredictable and can be dangerous for inexperienced swimmers.

Once you've found the pool, you're ready for a workout. A brief period of stretching can be helpful before you get into the pool. (You can use the basic flexibility exercises provided in chapter 6.) Once you're in the pool, warm up with slow strokes or kickboard work for about 5 to 10 minutes.

If your swimming workout is in a public pool, be courteous and watch out for others in the pool. Most pools have lanes divided to keep people from running into each other. More than two people can work out in a lane by swimming in an elongated circle (up one side—usually on the right—and back on the other). If only two of you are in a lane, you may want to "split" the lane, with each of you staying to one side. Often the lanes will be designated fast, medium, or slow. Swim in the lane that fits your speed. If you then find yourself passing people or being passed every few laps, look for a lane where the swimmers are closer to your own speed.

If your swimming workout lacks variety you can vary the distance, stroke, and intensity of your swims. To do this will take time: for beginners, about three to six weeks of two to three workouts per week. Initially, you will want to develop your endurance and stroke abilities so you can swim continuously for 15 to 20 minutes. Once you can swim continuously, you can increase the variety and aerobic training within your workout by varying the speed (see table 4.5). To vary your intensity, you might swim two laps faster and one lap slow, then repeat this cycle three to four times. Another way to vary your workout is to change strokes. Instead of swimming freestyle (crawl) or breaststroke, try alternating strokes between laps. By working on all four strokes—breaststroke, backstroke, butterfly, and freestyle—you not only make the workout more fun, but you also work different sets of muscles. You can also alter your workout by doing just the arm stroke (pulling) or just the leg stroke (kicking). For pulling, a foam rubber pull-buoy placed between your thighs will help keep your legs afloat and prevent you from kicking. If you want to work on kicking, use a kickboard.

Table 4.5 Sample Swimming Program

Week	Distance (meters)	Repetitions	Sets	Recovery	Total distance (meters)	Calories burned
			Low level*			
1	25	8	3	20 sec between reps; 1 min between sets**	600	160–180
2	25	8	3	15 sec between reps; 1 min between sets	600	160–200
3	25	10	3	15 sec between reps; 1 min between sets	750	180–220
4	25	12	3	15 sec between reps; 1 min between sets	900	200–240
Total weight lost: .88 pounds***						
5	50	2	3	15 sec between reps; 1 min between sets	900	200–260
	25	4				
	50	2				
6	50	3	3	15 sec between reps; 1 min between sets	1050	240–280
	25	2				
	50	3				
7	50	8	3	15 sec between reps; 1 min between sets	1200	260–300
8	50	8	3	10 sec between reps; 1 min between sets	1200	280–320
Total weight lost: 1.23 pounds						

*For all levels, the following specifications apply: 60–75% of HRmax, 6–8 calories burned per minute, RPE 12–13.

**During each workout, take heart rate during the 1-minute recovery between sets.

***Estimated weight loss in 4 weeks based on 4 swim workouts per week at an easy pace.

Week	Distance (meters)	Repetitions	Sets	Recovery	Total distance (meters)	Calories burned
Medium level						
1	25	3	4	15 sec between reps; 1 min between sets	1000	200–240
	50	2				
	75	1				
2	25	2	4	15 sec between reps; 1 min between sets	1100	220–260
	50	3				
	75	1				
3	25	3	4	15 sec between reps; 1 min between sets	1200	240–280
	50	3				
	75	1				
4	25	2	4	15 sec between reps; 1 min between sets	1200	260–300
	50	2				
	75	2				
Total weight lost: 1.12 pounds						
5	25	3	4	15 sec between reps; 1 min between sets	1300	270–310
	50	2				
	75	2				
6	25	3	4	15 sec between reps; 1 min between sets	1500	290–330
	50	3				
	75	2				
7	25	3	4	15 sec between reps; 1 min between sets	1600	300–340
	50	2				
	75	3				
8	25	3	4	15 sec between reps; 1 min between sets	1800	320–360
	50	3				
	75	3				
Total weight lost: 1.44 pounds						

(continued)

Table 4.5   (continued)

Week	Distance (meters)	Repetitions	Sets	Recovery	Total distance (meters)	Calories burned
				High level		
1	25	4	4	10 sec between reps; 1 min between sets	1250	210–280
	50	2				
	100	1				
2	25	2	4	10 sec between reps; 1 min between sets	1400	230–300
	50	2				
	100	2				
3	50	2	4	10 sec between reps; 1 min between sets	1400	230–300
	100	1				
	150	1				
4	50	3	4	10 sec between reps; 1 min between sets	1600	250–320
	100	1				
	150	1				
Total weight lost: 1.21 pounds						
5	50	4	4	10 sec between reps; 1 min between sets	1800	270–340
	100	1				
	150	1				
6	50	3	4	10 sec between reps; 1 min between sets	2000	290–360
	100	2				
	150	1				
7	100	2	4	10 sec between reps; 1 min between sets	2000	290–360
	150	2				
8	100	2	4	10 sec between reps; 1 min between sets	2200	310–380
	150	1				
	200	1				
Total weight lost: 1.45 pounds						

Hand paddles are another tool for improving your swimming strength and technique. The surface of the paddles is flat and smooth, so you need to place your hands properly during your pull. Hand paddles put an additional strain on your arms and shoulders, so they should not be used until you're in good condition. There are varying sizes of paddles and it's best to begin with paddles that are no bigger than your hand. Larger paddles can be used when you can easily handle the increased load on your arms and shoulders.

Once you become fit, you may want to try a more intense form of varied-speed training called *interval training*. This consists of swimming a set distance within a specified time interval. For example, a fast swimmer might swim 100 yards every 1 1/2 to 2 minutes and rest 15 to 40 seconds between each 100 yards. The distances and rest periods will depend on your capabilities, but generally the rest period should not be more than half of the swimming period. Depending on whether your goal is speed or endurance, the intervals can vary from 30 seconds (for 25-yard sprints) to 10 minutes and the number of repetitions from 2 to 10. In general, the times within a set should decrease only slightly (no more than 10 percent) from first to last.

Similar to the walking, running, and cycling programs, select your initial and subsequent training programs (in table 4.5) based on your fitness assessment results. We have not provided a swimming fitness assessment test, so you will need to base your swimming program on results obtained from either walking, running, or cycling fitness tests.

If you find that you really enjoy swimming, an excellent source of information on improving your swimming skills is *Fitness Swimming*, by Emmett Hines (1999). Swimming requires a specific skill-set, which is explained in detail in this book, along with over a year's worth of swimming workouts.

Water Exercises

In addition to swimming laps, you may want to consider other forms of water exercise, or "water aerobics." This form of exercise is great for those who want to enjoy the benefits of being buoyant in the water without having to swim. Some facilities offer 30- to 60-minute programs led by experienced water aerobics instructors. Even if you are a below-average swimmer (like me!) you can enjoy water aerobics and achieve the same fitness benefits.

Other pool exercises include water walking and running. Walking in shallow water adds resistance to walking and can strengthen your lower legs. Running in deeper water with a flotation vest allows you to do running movements in the pool without the restraints of pounding on your legs. This makes water exercises especially attractive to those with chronic arthritis. Usually water walking and jogging are done in two- to four-minute intervals with one- to two-minute rest periods. As most water exercise programs are not quite as intuitive as walking and jogging, you should seek out the advice of an experienced instructor before adding water aerobics or water exercises to your program.

Participating in Skill and Team Sports

Playing team sports is another very popular form of regular exercise. Team sports are a great way to combine exercise with socializing and will satisfy those competitive urges. Keep in mind that precision workload and heart rate targets are very difficult to measure while playing team sports; however, a brief pause in activity can allow you to measure your heart rate. Most sports require short bursts of activity (for example, a full-court basketball game), so wide swings in heart rate increase and recovery will occur.

You can measure your sport's intensity using METs. Refer to the table of MET values for common activities (table 4.1, page 59) or the Web site mentioned earlier in the chapter. A game of hoops (6 to 8 METs), field hockey (8 METs), or judo (13 METs) might be out of the question for you to do for 20 to 30 minutes as a part of your routine, so let's start out with walking (3 to 5 METs), table tennis (4 METs), or square dancing (3 to 7 METs).

To estimate the amount of calories you are burning running up and down a basketball court, do the following:

- Locate your sport in the MET table.
- Locate the energy cost in METs of your sport.
- Time how long you play.
- Multiply your weight (in kilograms) by the METs to estimate your calories burned per hour.
- If you played less than 60 minutes, divide the hourly rate by 60 and multiply that number (calories per minute) by the number of minutes you played.

Keep in mind that the 10 percent rule applies to sports play as much as walking, running, or biking. Do not increase your training by more than 10 percent per week. This includes your training intensity, the time for each workout, or the amount of calories you burn in a week of exercise. Why? Your risk of an overuse injury goes up if you increase training volume above 10 percent per week. An overuse injury early in the training program can force you to stop your program, taking you out of contention to control your blood pressure without medication. Remember, in the initial portion of your training routine, adding one extra workout per week will exceed the 10 percent rule. This is why we reduce the workload the week before we increase the number of workouts per week, or we don't increase until your weekly calorie burning is high enough to tolerate another workout.

It's Only a Game!

Here are some general rules for participating in team sports if you have high blood pressure.

▸ Remember, it's only a game. Don't let your temper get the best of you.

▸ Warm up and cool down gradually before and after games.

▸ Practice your sport-specific skills often.

▸ Remember, it's only a game.

▸ Game play should be only a portion of your total fitness program.

▸ Work on strength and flexibility exercises specific for the sport.

▸ Pain that lasts longer than two to three days should be evaluated by a sports physician.

▸ Remember, it's only a game.

Golf and bowling.   Let's be perfectly clear. Unless you walk the golf course, your blood pressure will probably not be reduced if golf is your only form of exercise during the week. (The one exception would be if golf is, for you, a form of stress management.) The aerobic benefits of playing golf will be limited to how far and fast you walk and how much your bag weighs. So if your passion for the game drives you to play often, walk whenever possible instead of riding in the cart. Another suggestion is to mix in flexibility and strength training for the trunk. If not done in conjunction with other forms of strength training and flexibility, golfers can develop muscle imbalances in the trunk and back that lead to more chronic low-back problems, resulting in pain when you do try to exercise. Core stability programs for golfers are an excellent way to supplement your game with the necessary strength, flexibility, coordination, and balance that will ultimately help your game.

Unless you are really unfit, taking three or four steps and hurling an 8-pound object down a waxed lane is not going to be enough strenuous activity to improve your blood pressure. And in most cases, playing the 10-pin is associated with other recreational consumption activities that tend to raise your blood pressure. If you enjoy bowling and your blood pressure is high, please do not use bowling as your only form of exercise. As in golf, trunk strength and flexibility will improve your game. Most people would receive more aerobic benefit from mowing the lawn—so do that or something else from the aerobic activity list before you head to the alley.

Choosing Exercise Specifics

One of the most important aspects of an effective exercise program is planning. Your plan should make it easy to exercise in terms of time, location, and facilities. Accounting for details such as where to exercise, what to wear, and how to prevent injuries will help your program to run smoothly and will prevent you from having problems that cause your program to stop. Here are some considerations specific to aerobic exercise.

Location

The exercise program can be difficult enough, so do what you can to make it easy on yourself to get to the gym, the workout room, or the walking path. Gyms should be close to home or to work. Home gyms should be in a separate designated area of the home that is a pleasant place to go into. Take your music, headphones, and water. Take something to read if you'll be exercising on the elliptical machine, treadmill, or stationary cycle. Exercising outdoors has its own set of factors to consider.

Indoor Exercise

Many will choose to begin their exercise program at the local gym. The indoor protection from the elements, the regular social environment, and a variety of exercise choices attract many to indoor facilities. For many, an easily accessible gym is all that is needed. Facility costs have become more affordable and hours have been expanded to make gym membership more practical for most. Some facilities provide childcare or children's activity programs, which certainly helps parents maintain a regular fitness program.

The variety of exercise activities is what attracts many to indoor exercise facilities. From treadmills to stair-climbing machines to rock-climbing walls, most indoor facilities pride themselves on providing a variety of safe, well-maintained exercise equipment. Almost all gyms provide not only aerobic conditioning exercise equipment but strength-training equipment as well. For many, gym membership is the only way to afford access to enough strength-training equipment to give an adequate workout. Many gyms also have a pool. Several employers who recognize the importance of a physically fit workforce have either added onsite gyms or arranged discounted gym memberships for their employees.

Most indoor aerobic exercise machines have the capability to accurately regulate your exercise intensity by controlling the speed, grade, or resistance of your activity. Many also have built-in heart rate monitors or have a heart rate monitor plug-in. Stair-climbing machines and cross-country ski machines are pieces of equipment that have been present in gyms for years. Stair-climbing machines offer a lower-impact form of climbing

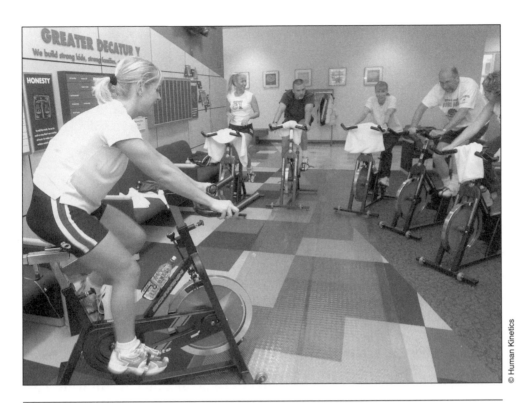

© Human Kinetics

Indoor fitness facilities offer many types of exercise equipment and modes, including group fitness classes, which many prefer for the social aspect.

exercise than running up stairs. Cross-country skiing requires the highest oxygen demand of any other form of aerobic exercise because the arms are used as much as the legs to cut through the snow. Cross-country skiing machines offer an excellent low-impact form of aerobic conditioning; some have been designed and priced for home use. Elliptical machines combine running, stair climbing, and cross-country skiing and are a very good form of low-impact exercise. Indoor rowers are an excellent and potentially addictive form of indoor training. Rowing offers a great total-body exercise as the upper body and back and legs are worked hard with little impact. The Concept-2 rower has been a solid fitness product for years for use in the gym or at home. Several indoor rowing workouts can be found at www.concept2.com/default.asp.

One word of caution: Before you purchase any type of home exercise equipment, try it out, use it regularly, and *really like it* for at least three months before you buy a similar piece of equipment for home use. Otherwise, you may find that your purchase will become the most expensive clothes rack you own.

Outdoor Exercise

If you choose to exercise outdoors, be safe. Above all, make your personal safety your priority. If you exercise outside, try to go with a buddy. Always be aware of your surroundings, and try not to exercise in an area that is completely foreign to you. Avoid late-night outdoor workouts and poorly lit areas. When traveling, try to stay in a motel that has indoor exercise facilities.

In most areas of the country, another concern with outdoor exercise is air quality. People with respiratory illnesses should avoid outdoor exercise when ozone levels are highest: at the end of the morning rush hour and during the afternoon rush hour. Ozone levels are usually highest during the summer months when heat and humidity are at their highest. Ozone also can accumulate to higher levels during cooler temperatures when there has been very little wind flow in an area for a few days. High ozone and poor air quality will cause breathing difficulties in those with respiratory disease but rarely cause significant problems (in the short term) for those who are disease free. Many communities will report on a daily basis the air quality index, which is a measure of both air pollution and ozone layers. Certainly, these levels vary by community and by the day, so it is important to be aware of how to find out the air quality before exercising outside if you have a respiratory illness. This includes those who have exercise-induced asthma and heart disease.

Scheduling

Many people ask when is the best time to exercise. The best time is when you have time. For most professionals, early morning, before the unpredictable demands of work kick in, is probably the best time. Many prefer the lunch hour, making their workout a well-deserved midday break. If you have time commitments, such as dropping off and picking up kids after school, the noon hour may be for you. Don't forget that a 15-minute walk at a break time during the day counts and can be as energizing as a cup of coffee or a power nap. Most are at their physiological best in the late afternoon and early evening hours. Runners, cyclists, weightlifters, and other athletes who track their workouts often claim more personal bests during afternoon or early evening workouts.

The times to avoid are those just before bed. A moderate-intensity workout has more of an energizing effect on the body than a relaxing effect and will disrupt sleep. A strenuous workout before sleep will require time to cool down and could not only disrupt sleep, but also prolong the onset of sound sleep. In addition, just as your mom always warned you not to swim until 30 minutes after you eat, it's best to avoid even moderate-intensity workouts in the first 30 to 60 minutes after a meal. On the other hand, a low-intensity, leisurely walk after a meal has no ill effects on either the exercising muscles or digestion and is probably a good idea to help burn off a few extra calories before they can go into storage around your waist and thighs.

If you're exercising outside, the temperature will probably dictate when you exercise more often than your schedule does. In order to avoid the effects of high temperatures and humidity, the best time to exercise is in the early evening. The next best time would be in the early morning; however, it is important to remember that this is usually the most humid time of the day, and your body's most efficient cooling mechanism, evaporation, will not work at its best. In colder climates, take advantage of the sun's warmth to exercise outside during the midday hours.

Exercise Apparel

Practically speaking, under- or overdressing for a workout can result in poor performance and the need to cut a workout short. Aerobic exercise takes the longest time to do, so above all dress comfortably.

Generated heat from burned calories must go away. Energy is neither created nor destroyed, so the energy used to move you along is transferred to the environment as heat. Even during exercise on the coldest days, body movement will always generate heat in direct proportion to the intensity and duration of the exercise. Your goal in selecting apparel should be to allow for an efficient transfer of heat in warm climates and to retain some heat in cold environments. It is always interesting to look over the field of a large running race that starts early in the morning during cooler temperatures. At the starting line, experienced runners are always the coldest because they know that once the race starts they will warm up quickly. The newbies are always the warmest and win the start line fashion contests. Unfortunately, those nice clothes usually find a new home later in the day, as they are shed on the race course to avoid the uncomfortable heat. Plastic garbage bags make great warm-ups! They tear away easy, cost very little, and are starting to come in attractive colors other than brown and black.

Cotton fabric absorbs best, but sweat will eventually accumulate into cotton clothing to the point of complete saturation, creating friction against the skin and preventing additional cooling. Some of the newer fabrics serve to wick away sweat from the skin to an outer layer, where the sweat is more easily evaporated. In cooler climates these fabrics are good base layers and can be covered by additional layers to help conserve heat while keeping chill-promoting sweat off the skin. In warm climates clothing that wicks sweat away from the skin is also a good option and can serve as the outermost layer. It is always tempting to expose as much skin as possible when exercising in a hot climate, and for cooling purposes this is ideal to promote evaporation. The radiant heat and UV radiation from the sun is well known to cause serious sunburns, so many appropriately cover themselves with skin lotions with sunblock. Some of the longer-lasting sunblocks, while providing adequate skin protection for longer periods, can disrupt the cooling mechanism and trap heat. The best advice is to avoid exercise during the heat of the day, from 10:00 to 3:00, when the sun's potential damage is greatest. If this is your only option, shorten your sun exposure or use a water-based skin lotion and reapply often to help keep you cooler during exercise.

Injury Prevention

The greatest risk period for developing an injury is in the first few weeks of a new fitness program. One study showed that the highest rate of injuries in new marathon trainees occurred within the first eight weeks of the program (Chorley et al. 2003). The risk increased again as new elements were added to the training program: speed work, hills, or more distance. As we've discussed, to avoid injury, experts recommend not increasing your exercise dosage more than 10 percent per week, whether you are a rookie or a veteran elite athlete. Also, guard those areas in which you have had a previous injury.

The other consistent risk factor for injury is a history of injury in the same area. On the flip side, a recently debunked tradition of stretching before exercise has been shown to be ineffective in preventing injury during exercise. Sounds like heresy to some, but it is important to remember that a warm ("warmed-up") muscle is more compliant and less likely to be injured during the strain of sudden effort or stretch. So advice now is to warm up by doing a lower-intensity activity, not necessarily stretching, before taking on the hard stuff. More on proper stretching and its importance in the fitness program will be discussed in chapter 6 on flexibility training.

Summary

At this point, you have established a training program that should result in several beneficial effects. Within four to six weeks you should notice an improved tolerance to physical tasks that once made you tired. You will begin to lose weight and will continue to lose weight at the rate of about one half to three quarters of a pound per week, perhaps more if you incorporate the healthy eating principles found in chapter 7. Above all, you will soon begin to feel better physically and feel better about yourself, and you will have made a significant step toward conquering your elevated blood pressure. Congratulations and keep going!

REGULATING PRESSURE THROUGH AEROBIC ACTIVITY

☐ Determine the appropriate "dosage" of aerobic exercise for blood pressure control:

- 30 to 60 minutes
- Three to five days a week
- 40 to 60 percent of maximum functional capacity

☐ Learn three ways to measure intensity:

- Metabolic equivalents (METs)
- Heart rate measurements
- Perceived exertion

☐ Choose from sample programs for walking, running, cycling, and swimming. Use the programs as they are, or customize one to your preferences and fitness level.

☐ Learn how to calculate exercise intensity for skill and team sports.

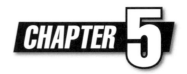
STRENGTHENING YOUR MUSCLES

A t least one of the motivating factors to exercise is to improve one's appearance, because we all know that when you look good, you feel good. When most of us think of exercise programs that help us to look good, we think of strength-training exercises. While it's true that strength training tones your muscles and gives them a pleasing appearance, and that this is a reasonable exercise goal, strength training also offers more important benefits for overall health—including improving blood pressure. The benefits of strength training are numerous. Larger, stronger muscles move more efficiently, more quickly, and with improved coordination. Stronger muscles are less likely to fail under the strain of lifting a moderately heavy load. Stronger muscles improve posture and act as shock absorbers across our joints, adding an additional layer of protection against excessive, arthritis-inducing shock to the joints. Strength training, if done properly, can improve muscle endurance and flexibility. Because of these many benefits, all people who exercise should include some form of strength training in their regular routines. This should be based on individual goals, health, and resources. When done correctly and safely, strength training is good for you.

Some commonly held myths and misconceptions about strength, strength training, and its place in a regular exercise program exist, and we will debunk those myths in this chapter. But first, let's look at how exactly strength training affects blood pressure.

How Strength Training Affects Blood Pressure

As discussed in chapter 2, there have been some misconceptions in the past about strength training possibly increasing blood pressure. A large analysis of several studies on resistance training reported a systolic and diastolic blood pressure reduction of 3 mmHg, or 2 to 4 percent, for those with normal pressures and with hypertension (Kelley and Kelley 2000). In addition, combining resistance and aerobic training results in an additive effect on blood pressure reduction.

Increased muscular strength results in the ability to improve movement efficiency, increase power, and improve neuromuscular coordination. All of these effects contribute to more efficient movement and, more than likely, to the lower resting blood pressure associated with training. Another potential factor is increased capillary density in growing muscles, which helps lower total peripheral resistance (TPR). Similar to aerobic training, resistance training can also result in a reduction in stress hormones, which also contributes to a lower TPR.

You do need to be cautious when straining to lift anything or when doing resistance training. When the body is involved in maximum or near-maximum lifts or contractions, the body involuntarily expands the chest, contracts the diaphragm, and contracts the trunk and back muscles. We hold our breath. This is done to keep our internal organs from shooting across the room when lifting a heavy object. Unfortunately, this maneuver, called the Valsalva maneuver, affects the return of blood back to the heart due to increased intra-abdominal and thoracic pressure. Thus, the flow of blood back to the heart is slowed to a halt, resulting in increases in pressure in the extremities—the blood has difficulty returning to the heart because of the high chest pressure created. As you might imagine, a slower return of blood to the heart means less blood is pumped out of the heart back to the body, and, most important, less blood will flow back to the brain. The brain is stingy—it likes blood flow. If it senses low flow, it says "no more" and shuts the system down until the contraction stops. This results in dizziness, or in fainting in an extreme condition. One way or the other, either by passing out or stopping the contraction, your brain is going to have its way and the flow of blood will return to normal.

The pressure changes brought about by the Valsalva maneuver are temporary, but it has nevertheless been believed that regular strength training would chronically increase blood pressure. Recent research again argues that this is not true, and in fact that the opposite probably occurs. If done correctly, regular strength training lowers blood pressure. It would be safer to avoid maximum lifts or extensive isometric exercise.

Common Strength Training Myths

In addition to the myth that strength training raises blood pressure in a negative way, there are other misconceptions about strength training that have been perpetuated through the years. It's important to know the truth so that you can take full advantage of the benefits strength training has to offer.

"I will look like one of those massive weightlifters if I lift weights."   Yes, probably so, if you train the way a competitive weightlifter trains. Athletes involved in the sport of weightlifting lift tons during each daily workout. But just as you probably will not look like an elite distance runner if you jog to the bakery daily, you probably will not look like an Olympic weightlifter if you add a few strength workouts to your exercise schedule.

"I only want to become toned; I don't want to get any bigger."   Usually, it's women who express this fear. But the majority of women will not become bigger by adding two or three strength workouts to their weekly routine; they will become more toned because the neuromuscular groups involved in the training routine will adapt to the workout. In addition, because you burn calories during strength-training workouts, you will lose fat weight if your training is complemented by an appropriate diet. Again, you will look like an elite bodybuilder only if you train the way an elite bodybuilder does and you have picked the right parents.

Most of us are not genetically blessed with an abundance of anabolic hormones, especially as we age. These hormones help to speed up the recovery process after a workout, thus allowing more work to be done in a shorter period. More work equals more potential for muscle adaptation and growth. More growth equals . . . well, you get the picture. This is why many have used supplemental anabolic hormones and steroids over the years—to allow them to recover quickly, to train harder, and to become bigger. Because most people do not have a natural abundance of these hormones, and because the amounts decrease as we age, they are not something to worry about if you're concerned about getting too big.

"I want to become bigger, so anabolic agents are a good choice—they won't hurt me."   This is a very bad choice for those who already have high blood pressure, high cholesterol, or prostate disease. Anabolic steroids will worsen each of these conditions and create a risk of developing other conditions, including heart disease and cancer. It's also a bad choice if you are a competitive athlete because almost every major sport governing body has a policy against the use of anabolic steroids and a testing program in place for detection of use as well as penalties for testing positive. Both male and female anabolic steroid users can develop male-pattern baldness, acne, mood swings, irritability, and depression. There has even been evidence that anabolic steroid use can become both psychologically and physically addictive. To use anabolic steroids is a potentially harmful choice with few long-term benefits and many potential risks. Don't do it.

"Weight training makes you stiff and inflexible."   If done correctly, strength training can actually improve flexibility. That "pumped-up" feeling you have after working out (and some seem to carry around with them all the time) is due to the temporary dramatic increase in blood flow to the exercised muscle, creating a feeling of fullness and inflexibility. In addition, the well-exercised muscle is significantly fatigued, which can limit contraction throughout the normal full range of motion. Once this "pump" is gone, the flexibility of the muscle or its ability to move efficiently throughout a full range of motion returns to normal. This book also provides flexibility exercises, and we strongly recommend adding these to your workouts to further maintain flexible muscles.

"I've never lifted weights before and I'm afraid I'll pull a muscle." Yes, it is possible to pull a muscle when lifting weights, especially if performing a technique incorrectly. It is also possible to pull a muscle moving the furniture, picking up your kids or grandkids, washing the car, or even getting up off the couch. If you add resistance to any movement and you are unaccustomed to added resistance, your muscle can overextend itself and become sore, pulled, or otherwise injured. When done properly, strength training will reduce the chances of muscle injury when performing activities of daily living, again because the muscle units are more toned, stronger, and more efficient at recruiting other muscle groups to help if the resistance is too great. Regular strength training will accomplish two purposes: first, the resistance used for appropriate strength-training exercises will be enough to promote adaptation but not enough to result in acute injury. Second, if you strength train regularly, you will know your limits and how much weight you can safely lift.

"I'm a runner, so I don't need to do weight training for my legs." Strength-training exercises for the hips and legs of runners, cyclists, walkers, and others who do most of their aerobic conditioning upright is more important than upper-body strength training. Strength exercises for the hamstrings, glutes, and groin area have been shown in a few studies to help reduce overuse injuries, such as iliotibial band syndrome, knee pain, and back pain, in endurance athletes (Fredericson et al. 2000). Runners need only to mix in a couple of strength training sessions a week to reap the benefits.

"Weight training makes your muscles sore." Yes, this is true, especially if your training program involves a lot of eccentric or "negative" resistance exercises. A *negative,* or *eccentric,* contraction is one in which the muscle must contract while it is lengthening. Normally, a muscle shortens as it contracts. An example of an eccentric contraction is the contraction of the biceps while lowering a weight, or of the hamstrings when going into a squatting position. The eccentric contraction is as important as the concentric contraction of a movement because it helps in the movement by adding stability and strength. Without the eccentric component of most movements, our ability to move against resistance would be limited.

Getting back to the soreness issue, eccentric contraction results in microscopic damage to the muscle—damage that is temporary, easily repaired, and part of the normal process of recovery from exercise. If excessive, the recovery process will result in localized swelling, increasing the sense of stiffness and prolonging soreness. This feeling can last

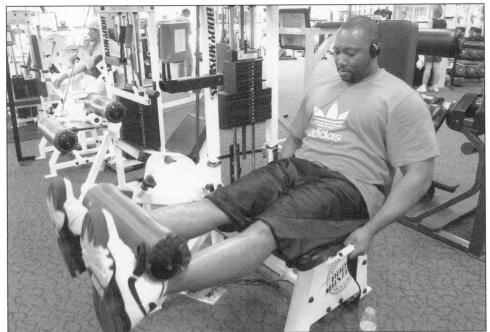

© Human Kinetics

Mild muscle soreness that results from strength training is a good thing—it means your muscles are rebuilding stronger after microscopic damage.

anywhere from 12 hours to 5 days after an activity, and the time of discomfort is directly related to the amount of exercise intensity. Oddly enough, movement improves the discomfort, so it is best to get back up on the "horse that made you sore." Ice, heat, massage, and over-the-counter medications have been found to temporarily relieve the discomfort of delayed-onset muscle soreness (DOMS). The best way to treat this is to ease gradually into strength training and to reduce the amount of eccentric contractions.

Proper Load and Progression

In order to make changes, increase in tone and size, move more efficiently, and adapt to training, the rested and recovered muscle must be repeatedly challenged to move against increasing resistance. All too often, people with the best intentions begin a program of exercise, do too much too soon, become sore or injured, and quit. Can't criticize that logic one bit. The best way to avoid dropping out is to plan ahead and pace yourself. Do not try to meet your initial fitness goals in three weeks or less—unless, of course, your goal is to have exercised every other day for those three weeks! To meet this compliance goal it is best to start slow and gradually increase.

How much resistance should be used? Start at a low level. In chapter 3 we determined your estimated one-repetition max lift (1RM) for the bench press and the leg press. The weights lifted in these two tests are usually 68 to 79 percent of your 1RM and are based on your level of training and weight-training experience (Braith et al. 1993). It is possible to check your 1RM for each individual lift (overhead press, leg curl, arm curl, pulldown, and so on) you intend to use during training, but this would take considerable time. An easy way to choose a beginner's weight is to assume that your 1RM for an upper- and lower-body exercise is about 50 percent of your 1RM bench and leg press weights. Multiply your submaximal test weights by 0.7 to get a beginning training weight. If you are using dumbbells, begin an upper-body lift with half of your beginning training weight. This should be a weight you can easily lift for 2 or 3 sets of 8 to 12 repetitions (as described later). This is a lot of "barbell math," but it is important to optimize your training program and lower the risk of training injury.

In order to improve tone and the ability to move efficiently against resistance, the body must adapt to increasingly heavier loads. This adaptation must be gradual and individual: there is no one ideal recommendation for progression that fits everyone. Progression is the art of exercise prescription. Again, at the beginning of a program the amount of weight lifted or resistance should be easy enough to perform at least 8 repetitions and hard enough that you become tired after 15 to 20 repetitions. As you progress, the weight or resistance increases yet is easy enough to lift 8 to 12 times and hard enough to result in fatigue after 15 to 20 repetitions. Starting out, you do only one set of 8 to 20 repetitions. When you can easily reach 20 repetitions, you should have recovered your energy enough to add an additional set of at least 8 repetitions. When you can do 3 sets of 20 repetitions, it's time to increase the weight lifted. Generally, this is about 5 to 10 pounds per exercise. This extra weight can be added during the next workout.

If you find that you are too sore after increasing the number of weights, repetitions, or sets, do not increase the weights, reps, or sets for the next workout. Soreness, especially during the initial phase, is normal, but the recovery process for soreness takes longer initially and improves as a part of the adaptation process. Therefore, take your time and do not progress until you are pain free.

Your body may not adapt to each exercise at the same speed. This is normal. In other words, you may be able to do 3 sets of exercises for your legs but only 2 sets for your upper body. This is OK, and by continuing to follow this plan, you will avoid injury and maximize your potential strength gains.

Just as with aerobic exercise, a good rule of thumb regardless of the form of training is to not increase your training volume (weight, repetitions, sets, and number of workouts per week) by more than 10 percent per week. Research shows that the rate of injury increases dramatically if training volume increases by more than 10 percent per week. The best way to avoid this is to go slow, especially during the initial phase of training. Another good way to avoid overtraining is to record your routine in an exercise log and compare from week to week.

Equipment and Location

When starting out your strength program, accurately assess your resources. Are you going to go to a gym, or are you going to use your kid's old barbells and weights in the basement? When you're starting out, make working out as easy and accessible as possible; otherwise it will be much easier when you're tired or a little sore to justify not going across town to the gym for your workout. In other words, keep it close. A gym at work or at home is probably the easiest and most accessible. Some type of initial financial investment has also been found to improve compliance with training—you will be less likely to drop out if you have put some money into it.

When starting out, the best equipment for home use is dumbbells. Pick out and purchase three or four pairs. When trying to decide how much weight to buy, take this book to the store with you and try out a few of the exercises in the dumbbell program. You should be able to easily do 15 to 20 repetitions for the exercise with the lowest weight you choose—for most, a beginning pair of 5- to 10-pound dumbbells can be used. If you have no experience with resistance training, select a 3-pound pair for starters. As you progress, you will need more resistance, so in addition to the lightest pair of dumbbells get two or three additional pairs, each about 5 pounds heavier than the next. Purchase the sturdiest types of dumbbells you can afford, because they can take a beating, and you don't want to abruptly end your program because of equipment failure. Once you have completed the first three cycles of the dumbbell program you can go back to the same store and buy heavier pairs or switch to using barbells or machines. Personally, I like the dumbbell program because it is easy, you can do it at home, and you build coordination by training both sides of the body independently.

Proper Strength-Training Technique

Here are a few general tips to use during your resistance workouts. If you're not following the training programs described here, always begin your workout doing exercises that use larger muscles first, such as the leg press, lunge, or squat. Then progress to exercises that use smaller muscle groups, such as the arm curl. This will reduce the possibility of not finishing a workout because you are too tired. Make sure when doing an exercise that you follow the proper form throughout the set. Never compromise your form to lift more weight. When in doubt, ask for help from an expert.

Proper breathing can add to the safety of resistance training for those with hypertension. Remember that holding your breath can result in an extreme rise in blood pressure! An easy breathing technique is to inhale during the easiest portion of the lift and exhale during the hardest. For example, on a squat or bench press, inhale when lowering the weight and exhale when pushing the weight back up.

As you become fatigued, the weights will be harder to hold. Make sure that you avoid holding weights above your head or face for a prolonged period of time near the end of a set. Injuries occur during weight training as a result of fatigue, so if you are fond of your teeth, and most of us are, keep those dumbbells away from your face on the eight, ninth, and tenth repetitions!

It is good to rest between sets. The ideal amount varies with your level of conditioning. Initially, try to take about 2 to 3 minutes between sets. As you get into better condition, you can shorten the rest period to 30 seconds between sets and benefit from additional gains in fitness. Shorter rest periods with higher-intensity resistance during exercise is often referred to as *interval training* and is a great way to increase your level of fitness.

Strength-Training Programs

Two types of workouts are provided here: one for upper- and lower-body strengthening, and one specifically for core stability training. The upper- and lower-body workout provides exercises for the major muscle groups, including arms, legs, back, and chest.

Core stability training is not new, but the benefits in terms of performance enhancement and injury prevention have been recently reported. The *core* simply refers to the trunk, both front and back. The idea of stability training emphasizes the principle that arms and legs work better from a stable trunk platform. The stable trunk is able to adapt to both changes in resistance and other ground forces that try to make the body unstable. Changing surfaces, positions, and loads all will "unbalance" the core and adversely affect movement. Core training emphasizes training the trunk to efficiently adapt to changing forces through a series of low-resistance moves done in different positions or on different surfaces. The result is improved balance and coordination, as well as a lower risk of the most common overuse injury: low-back pain. The benefits of core stability training are so great that it should be included in every exercise program. There is such a wide variety of exercises available that it is difficult to become bored with this type of training, even if it is done daily. The benefits are usually noticed quickly. There is little or no risk associated with this type of training, but the initial phase of the program should be supervised by someone knowledgeable in this form of training.

The sample programs included in this chapter are divided into three levels. They should seem easy when you start your program. They should be so easy that you want to keep doing them and have no problems coming back for the next workout. The sample program details are shown in tables 5.1, 5.2, and 5.3. The programs are made up of the upper- and lower-body workouts and the core training workouts. Remember that these programs are examples that you can use as they are or customize to better fit your specific strength level and needs. Specific exercise instructions and illustrations are given in the next section.

Table 5.1 Comprehensive Strength-Training Program—Low Level

Days	Workout focus	Exercises	Sets	Repetitions	Rest between sets
Week 1					
Monday, Wednesday	Upper and lower body	All 11 exercises*	1	10	2 minutes
Tuesday, Thursday	Core stability	All 8 exercises**	1	10	2 minutes
Week 2					
Monday, Wednesday	Upper and lower body	All 11 exercises	1	15	1 minute
Tuesday, Thursday	Core stability	All 8 exercises	1	15	1 minute
Week 3					
Monday, Wednesday	Upper and lower body	All 11 exercises	1	10	30 seconds
Tuesday, Thursday	Core stability	All 8 exercises	1	10	30 seconds
Week 4					
Monday, Wednesday	Upper and lower body	All 11 exercises	1	15	30 seconds
Tuesday, Thursday	Core stability	All 8 exercises	1	15	30 seconds

*Exercise instructions given on pages 95 through 105.

**Exercise instructions given on pages 106 through 113.

Table 5.2   Comprehensive Strength-Training Program—Medium Level

Days	Workout focus	Exercises	Sets	Repetitions	Rest between sets
Week 1					
Monday, Wednesday	Upper and lower body	All 11 exercises*	2	10	1 minute
Tuesday, Thursday	Core stability	All 8 exercises**	2	10	1 minute
Week 2					
Monday, Wednesday	Upper and lower body	All 11 exercises	2	15	1 minute
Tuesday, Thursday	Core stability	All 8 exercises	2	15	1 minute
Week 3					
Monday, Wednesday	Upper and lower body	All 11 exercises	2	10	30 seconds
Tuesday, Thursday	Core stability	All 8 exercises	2	10	30 seconds
Week 4					
Monday, Wednesday	Upper and lower body	All 11 exercises	2	15	30 seconds
Tuesday, Thursday	Core stability	All 8 exercises	2	15	30 seconds

*Exercise instructions given on pages 95 through 105.

**Exercise instructions given on pages 106 through 113.

If you have recent experience with resistance training, begin with the medium-level program. This "step-up" program allows you to do an extra set of each exercise with less rest between sets than in the low-level program. You will still only do resistance training for each muscle group twice a week. If you have access to and experience with resistance training machines, you may choose them as another way to strength train, instead of using dumbbells. The exercises are similar. Follow the same number of reps, sets, and rest between sets that you would follow for the dumbbell program.

If you have already been weight training regularly and have considerable experience, begin with the high-level program (you may also progress from the low, to the medium, to the advanced program as your training

Table 5.3 **Comprehensive Strength-Training Program—High Level**

Days	Workout focus	Exercises	Sets	Repetitions	Rest between sets
Week 1					
Monday, Wednesday, Friday	Upper and lower body	All 11 exercises*	3	10	1 minute
Tuesday, Thursday	Core stability	All 8 exercises**	3	10	1 minute
Week 2					
Monday, Wednesday, Friday	Upper and lower body	All 11 exercises	3	15	1 minute
Tuesday, Thursday	Core stability	All 8 exercises	3	15	1 minute
Week 3					
Monday, Wednesday, Friday	Upper and lower body	All 11 exercises	3	10	30 seconds
Tuesday, Thursday	Core stability	All 8 exercises	3	10	30 seconds
Week 4					
Monday, Wednesday, Friday	Upper and lower body	All 11 exercises	3	15	30 seconds
Tuesday, Thursday	Core stability	All 8 exercises	3	15	30 seconds

*Exercise instructions given on pages 95 through 105.

**Exercise instructions given on pages 106 through 113.

improves). This workout is a traditional, three-times-per-week program that also includes core training on the off days. With the advanced program you will be doing three sets of each exercise. Similar to the medium-level program, those with experience using resistance training machines can substitute machine training for dumbbells, following the same program. Those doing the advanced program may also have experience using a regular barbell. A long barbell may be substituted for dumbbells in this program.

One note on the programs: It's best to skip a day between strength training workouts to allow your muscles to rest and rebuild, and thus get stronger. In our program, we have you do exercises for the upper and lower body on Mondays and Wednesdays, then exercises for the core on Tuesdays and Thursdays. This follows the principle of skipping a day because you are not exercising the same area of the body two days in a row. You can change the days (for example, exercise on Saturday instead of one of the weekdays); just make sure you keep to this principle.

STANDING ROW

Stand with feet about shoulder-width apart. Bend forward at the waist and bend the knees slightly. Hold a dumbbell in each hand, with arms straight down toward the floor. Keeping the back straight, pull the dumbbells toward your chest until the upper arms are parallel to the floor. For added leg work, squat to the floor, allowing the weights to touch the floor. Then stand, waist bent and back straight, and complete the row.

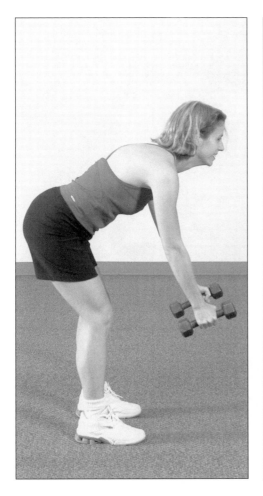
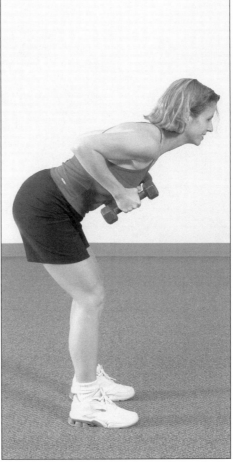

REVERSE BUTTERFLY

Holding a light dumbbell in each hand with arms toward the floor, lie facedown on a flat or incline bench and raise the dumbbells to your sides without bending your elbows. At the top of the movement, try to bring your shoulder blades together before lowering the weights back forward.

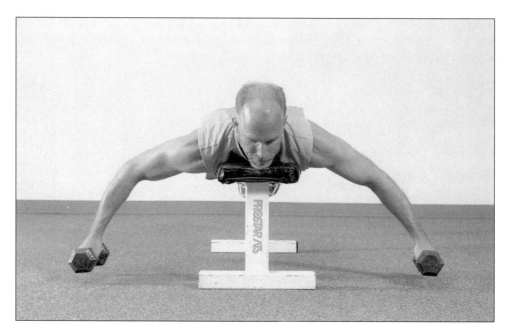

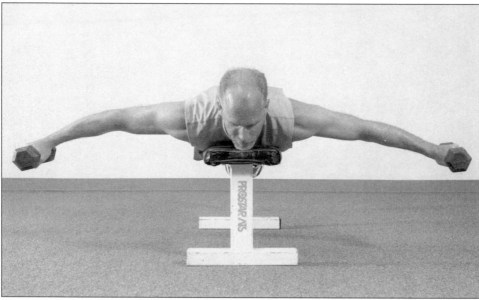

DUMBBELL BENCH PRESS

Lie on your back, holding dumbbells on your chest with palms facing toward the ceiling and elbows bent. Press the dumbbells up. Bring them back down to your sides. Note that when you use dumbbells instead of a barbell, a wider range of motion can be achieved by bringing the dumbbells to your sides instead of your chest.

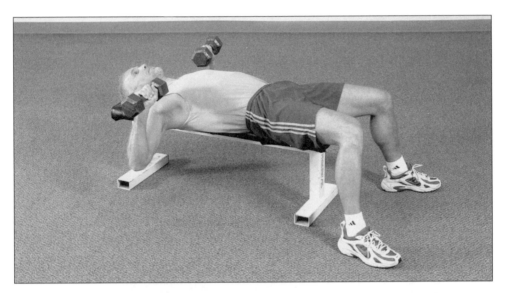

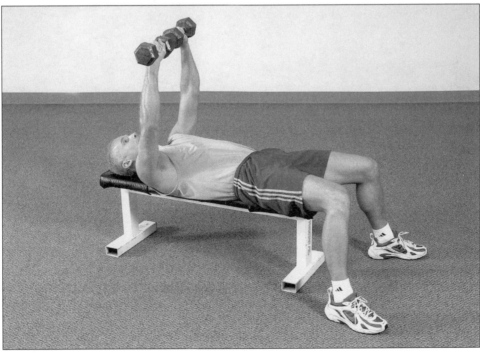

ARM CURL

Stand with feet about shoulder-width apart. With a light bar or dumbbells held at the waist, bend at the elbows and lift the weights to your chest. Bring the weights back to your waist.

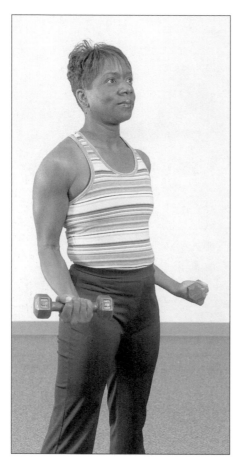 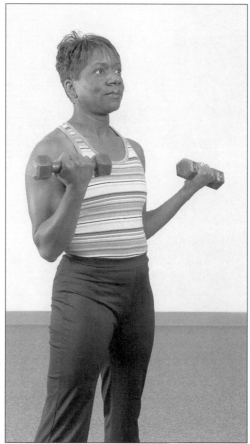

SEATED CLEAN AND PRESS

While seated on an incline bench, hold light dumbbells at your sides. Lift the weights to your shoulders, then press the weights overhead. Carefully lower the weights back to the start position.

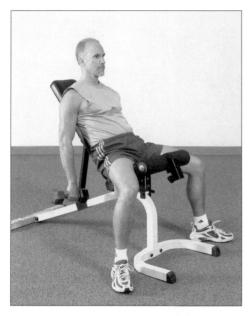 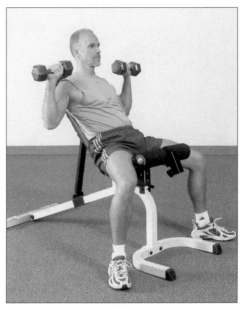

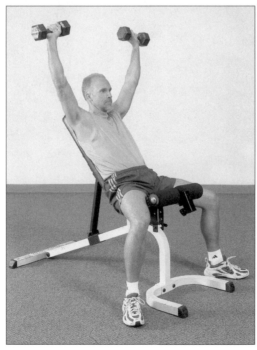

LUNGE

While standing, hold a light bar or broomstick behind your head. With alternating legs, step forward and bend at the knee with one leg and allow the opposite leg to bend and touch the floor. Push back up with the forward leg and repeat with the opposite leg stepping forward.

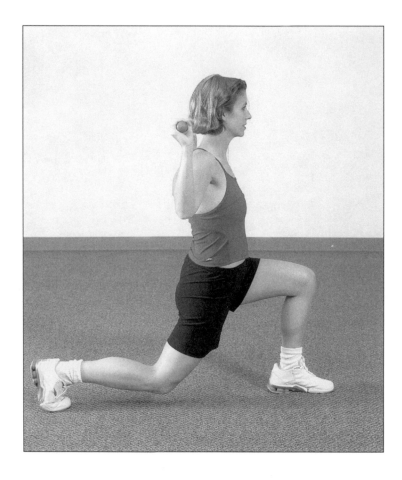

LEG EXTENSION

While seated, add resistance to your lower legs in the form of a weight or resistance band or with the help of a machine lever. From a bent start position, straighten or extend both legs. Lower the weight by carefully bending the knees.

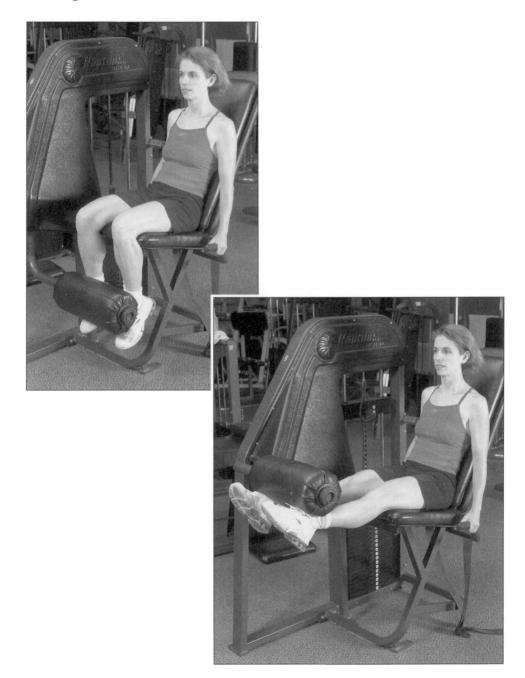

LEG CURL

Lie facedown on a resistance bench or floor. Start with the legs straight with resistance added at the ankles and lift the weight by bending at the knees. Return slowly to the start position.

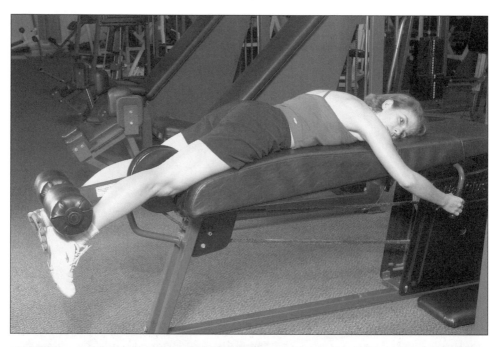

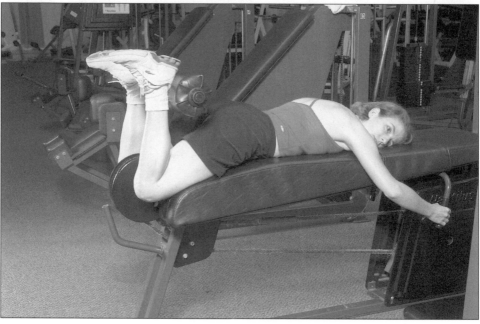

HIP EXTENSION AND HIP FLEXION

For hip extension, add resistance to the lower leg at the ankle—a resistance band works best. Stand facing the object the resistance band is fastened to. With both knees slightly bent, extend the leg with the resistance backward (see first photo). Unless you have a means to add resistance to both sides, do all the repetitions on one leg and then change the resistance to the opposite leg.

For hip flexion, use a resistance band as with hip extension. Stand facing away from the object the resistance band is fastened to. Extend the leg with the resistance forward (see second photo).

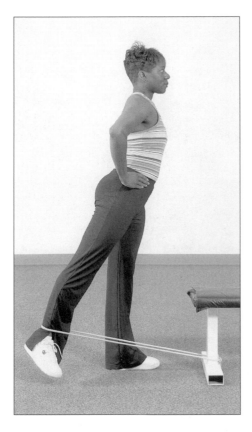
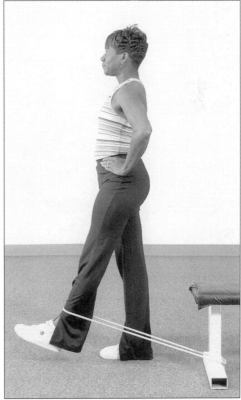

HIP ABDUCTION AND HIP ADDUCTION

For hip abduction, fasten a resistance band to the lower leg at the ankle. Stand sideways to the object the resistance band is fastened to, with the band on the leg farther from the object (the band will cross your other leg). With both knees slightly bent, extend the leg with the resistance to the side (see first photo). Unless you have a means to add resistance to both sides, do all the repetitions on one leg and then change the resistance to the opposite leg.

For hip adduction, use a resistance band as with hip abduction. Stand sideways to the object the resistance band is fastened to, with the band on the leg closer to the object. Bring the leg with the resistance across the other leg (see the second photo).

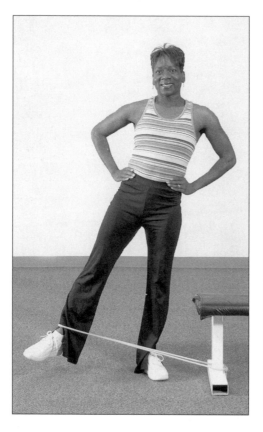 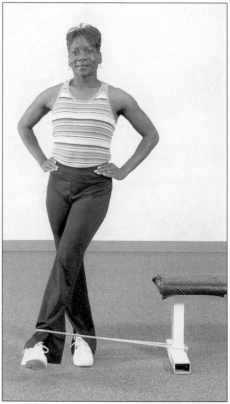

LEG PRESS

On a leg press resistance machine, adjust the seat with help from an instructor. With lower weight, lower the resistance "sled" with the legs until the knees are bent beyond 90 degrees. Push the sled forward until the legs are extended.

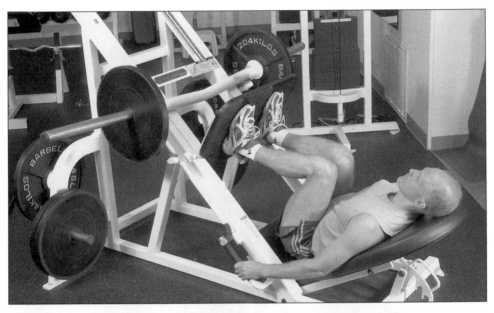

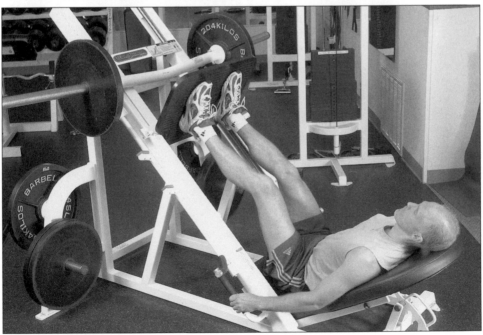

WALL SQUAT

While standing against a door or wall, squat down and stand back up with the wall supporting your back. For more fun, squeeze a ball between your knees.

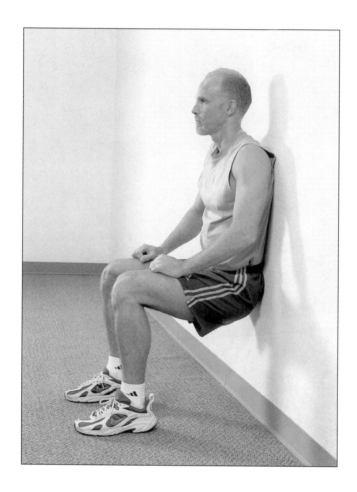

SINGLE-LEG SQUAT

This can be done against a wall or not. Squat down on one leg and stand up. Try to avoid allowing the knee to bend inward ("bowlegged") while squatting or standing.

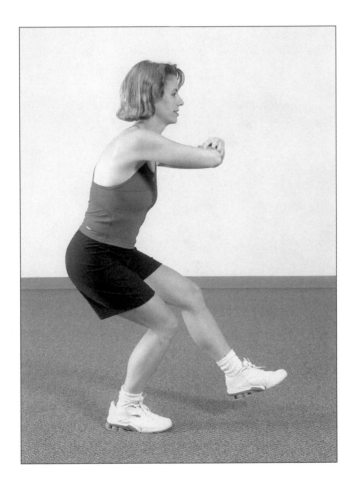

STANDING ABDUCTOR

From a balanced stand, raise one leg to the side while balancing on the opposite leg. Hold your arms out to your sides to help you balance. Alternate legs.

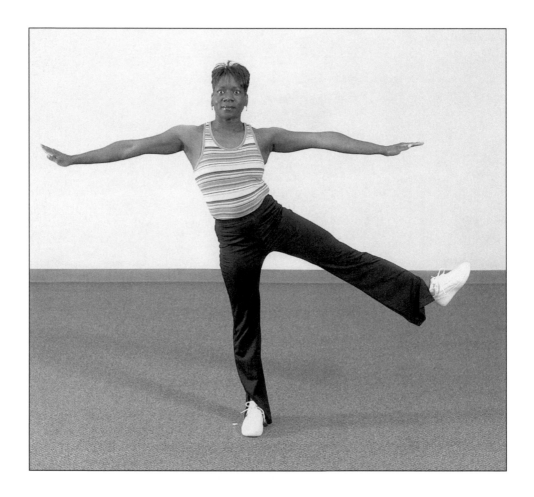

PRONE ABDUCTOR

Kneel on all fours. Raise one leg to the side, with the knee bent. Return to the start position. Repeat with the other leg.

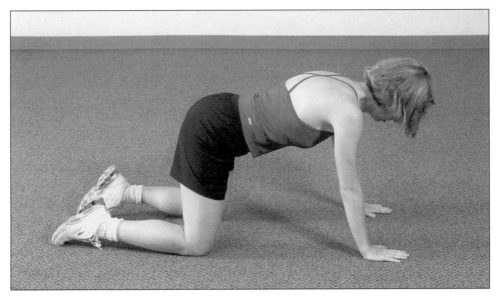

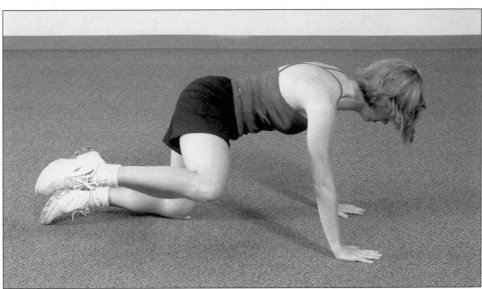

STANDING X-MAN

While standing, extend one leg backward and extend the opposite arm forward while balancing on the opposite leg. Beginners should be able to do this exercise lying facedown before attempting it while standing.

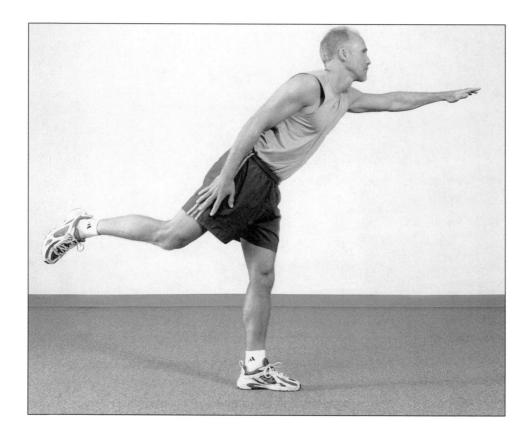

DONKEY KICK

Kneel on all fours. Kick one leg straight back, then return to the start position. Alternate kicking legs. For advanced work, raise the opposite arm at the same time as you kick.

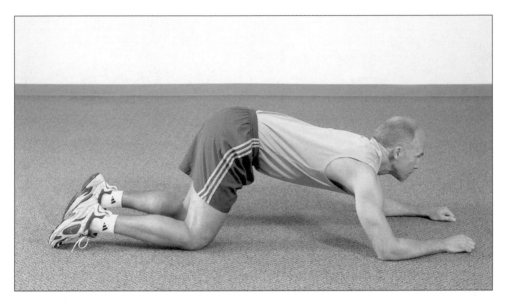

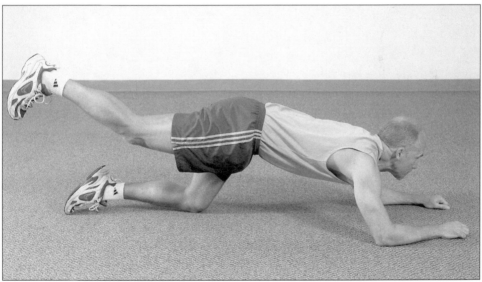

SIDE KICK

While lying on your side, place one leg forward and the other behind you with both knees straight. Alternate raising your forward and backward legs. After one set, don't forget to lie on the other side and repeat.

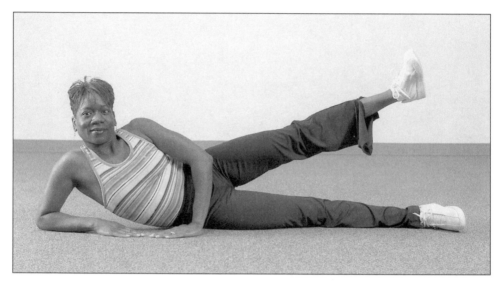

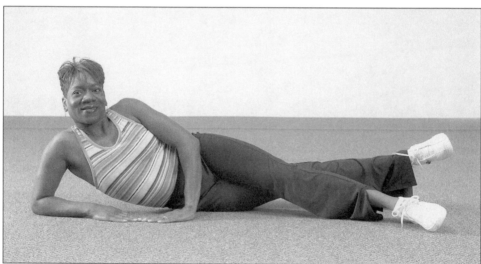

LAWNMOWER STARTER

Stand with the legs more than shoulder-width apart and bend at the waist and knees, touching the opposite foot. In an angular fashion raise the arm across your body and then overhead, using the same motion as pulling a mower cord. Repeat using the opposite arm.

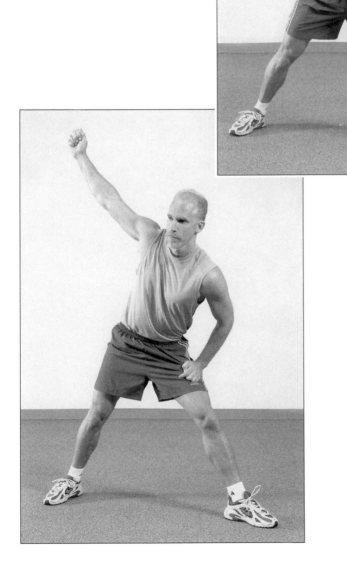

Summary

Don't you feel stronger already? Seriously, gains in strength from resistance training come rapidly. In fact, the most rapid gain of strength is in the first four to six weeks of a strength-training program. This is probably because of the learning, or improved lifting coordination, effect. Nonetheless, you will see some of the most noticeable gains with this form of training. Once you have reached a plateau, stay with it, gradually increase your resistance level, or shorten the time between sets. An effective strength-training program is yet another way to take control of the management of your blood pressure.

ACTION PLAN:

STRENGTHENING YOUR MUSCLES

☐ Learn the truth behind several common myths about strength training.

☐ Determine how much weight to start with based on your current strength, and how to progress from there.

☐ Ensure proper weightlifting technique to reduce problems or risk of injury.

☐ Use the sample strength programs provided, or customize them to fit your preferences and needs.

☐ Take advantage of the 19 exercises described and illustrated.

CHAPTER 6

GAINING AND MAINTAINING FLEXIBILITY

Flexibility, balance, and strength can be gained by adding a core stabilization program to your regimen. What exactly is flexibility? For years we equated being able to touch your toes with being "flexible" or "in shape." Simply, flexibility is the elasticity, or stretchability, of a muscle group. Some of us are tight, some loose, most in between.

Unlike the evidence for aerobic and resistance exercise, there is very little evidence to support the use of flexibility training as a means to control blood pressure. A few smaller studies support the notion that the regular practice of tai chi or yoga has a positive impact on blood pressure (Lee 2004). Although these are small studies, it makes intuitive sense that performing these exercise routines daily as a form of relaxation therapy could improve blood pressure via stress reduction. The improvement in flexibility (along with mild improvements in both aerobic capacity and strength) would be secondary gains.

Why is flexibility important? Again, for years it has been thought that the more flexible the muscles are, the less likely they are to be injured. This is most likely true, as the compliance of a muscle does tend to improve with stretching. However, because the muscle is attached to a joint, or crosses a joint, a more flexible muscle can result in injury in some cases. For example, the muscles of the shoulder must have a delicate balance of flexibility, strength, and stability, or the shoulder will dislocate. If the muscles were too tight you would not be able to execute basic motions, such as to raise your arm overhead, throw a ball, use a tennis racket, or comb your hair. The same can be said of the kneecap area (patella), ankle, and hip. In other words, flexible muscles are good, and are probably less likely to be injured, but muscle groups must work together and function in a coordinated fashion to balance stability and flexibility to avoid injury.

There are at least three areas of the body in which being flexible is important for well-being, and they are generally the tightest: the lower back, hamstrings, and hip flexors. These muscles contribute to the body's core strength as well as flexibility. Inflexibility of these three muscle groups more than likely is a major contributor to most low-back problems. Because this is such a common problem, we will focus on these areas for flexibility training. Other areas that will receive less emphasis are areas that are problematic for fewer people. They include the neck and upper-back muscles, the quadriceps, and the calves. These areas can also contribute to tightness and, in some people, chronic pain, often in the neck.

Time, Frequency, and Technique

Flexibility training should be done daily. There is controversy at present as to when to do stretching exercises in relation to other exercises. Traditionally, stretching has been included in the warm-up portion of aerobic or strength exercise sessions as a means of preventing injury. Currently there is no good data to support the notion that muscle injuries are prevented if stretching is done as part of a regular warm-up. In fact, basic muscle physiology dictates that a warm muscle is more compliant and hence more "stretchable." So stretching a cold muscle can actually cause muscle injury. With this idea in mind, this program recommends that warm-up exercises consist of just that: warming up. The best way to do this is to start your main exercise mode slowly (walking, running, cycling) and gradually increase the intensity of exercise or to do low-intensity calisthenic exercises, such as jumping jacks and toe touches. The flexibility program will then follow the aerobic portion, as the muscles should be sufficiently warm and stretched following a workout.

There are many techniques for doing flexibility exercises. I recommend *not* doing ballistic stretches—those with repetitive bouncing motions. This program emphasizes static stretching techniques: establishing a position stretching the muscle and holding that position for a count of 10, releasing, and then repeating for another 10 count. People who have low muscle flexibility may benefit from doing these exercises daily. Combining a few flexibility exercises with a basic set of core strength exercises creates a workout time commitment of only about 10 minutes. Remember, if you don't do a full warm-up or aerobic exercise session before flexibility training, you must be much more careful and may find that you obtain less range of motion than when you are warm. An exercise tip: Wear comfortable clothing and do a few jumping jacks or toe touches or jog in place for a couple of minutes before stretching to warm up.

The Flexible 10

Warm the body by doing gradual, slow, nonjerking calisthenic motions, such as toe touches, side bends, lunges, or overhead reaching. You can also add a low-intensity walk, jog, bike ride, or other aerobic activity before beginning the following flexibility exercises. The core strength exercises described in the previous section may also be used as a muscle warm-up. The 10 flexibility exercises described in this section focus on improving flexibility in the main problem areas. Follow the technique guidelines given in the previous section when performing these stretches. If you do these exercises correctly, you will also receive added stress reduction from your daily flexibility routine.

WALL PUSH CALF STRETCH

Stretches the calves

Stand facing a wall or firm object, keeping one or both legs straight at the knee, feet shoulder-width apart. Lean forward, catching yourself with either your hands or forearms leaning against the wall, until you feel a stretch in your lower legs.

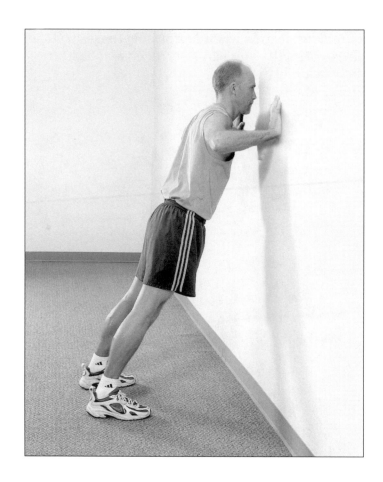

FLAMINGO STRETCH

Stretches the quadriceps and hip flexors

Facing a wall, bend the right leg backward and pull the foot toward your buttocks with your right hand. Repeat with the left leg. For additional stretching, lean forward against the wall. If necessary, use one hand to support yourself against the wall.

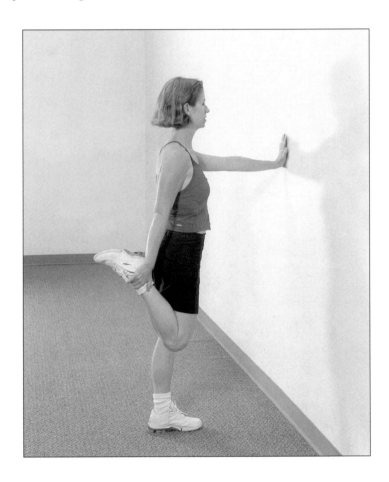

KNEELING LUNGE

Stretches the hip flexors

From a kneeling position, step forward (lunge) with one leg, keeping the opposite leg kneeling on the floor. Leaning forward will further stretch the usually tight hip flexors.

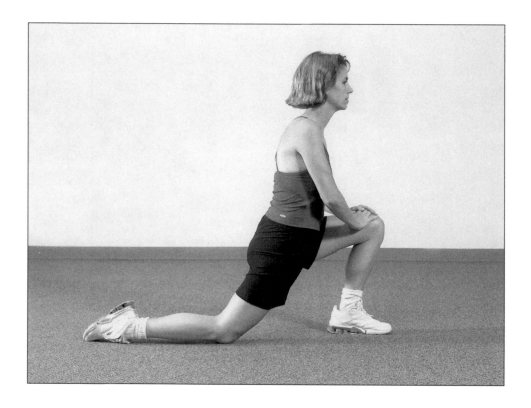

BUTTERFLY STRETCH

Stretches the thigh adductors

While seated, bend the knees and bring the feet toward the crotch as far as possible. Push against the inside of the knees with the elbows and hold.

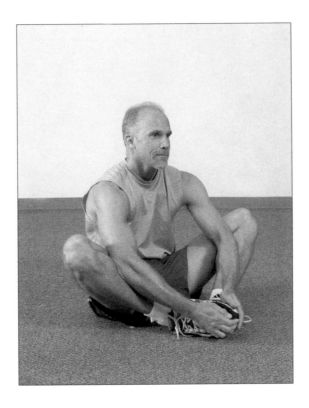

PELVIC TILT

Stretches the lower-back muscles

While lying on your back, bend your knees and place your feet on the floor or on a stool. In this position, roll and tilt the pelvis forward by pushing your belly button toward the floor and flattening the lower back against the floor.

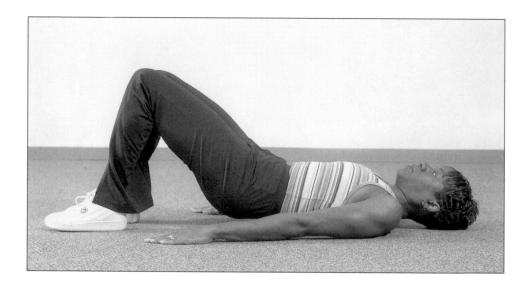

KNEE TO CHEST STRETCH

Stretches the hamstrings, glutes, and low back

While lying on your back, bend one knee and pull it toward your chest. You can keep a slight bend in your opposite knee for comfort. Try to maintain the pelvic tilt and flat back from the previous stretch. Repeat with the opposite leg.

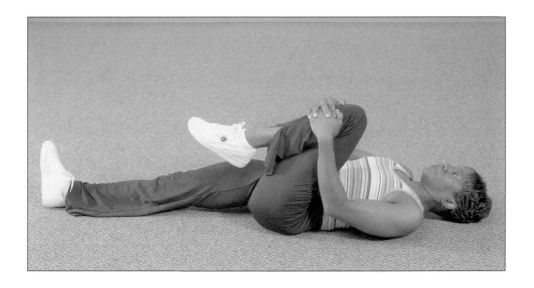

MODIFIED HURDLER STRETCH

Stretches the calves, hamstrings, glutes, and low back

While seated, extend one leg straight forward and bend the opposite leg at the knee, bringing the foot toward the crotch. Lean forward over the straight leg and hold.

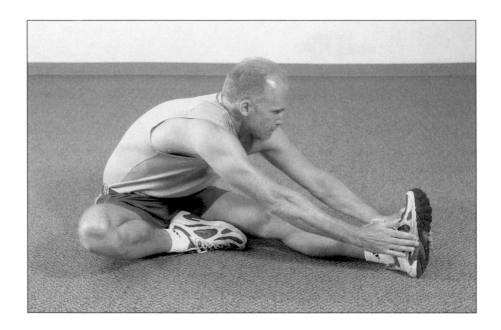

FIGURE 4

Stretches the low back and trunk rotators

While lying on your back keep one leg straight, bend the opposite leg, and hook the foot of the bent leg behind the straight knee. Roll the trunk toward the side of the straight leg until the bent knee touches the floor and hold.

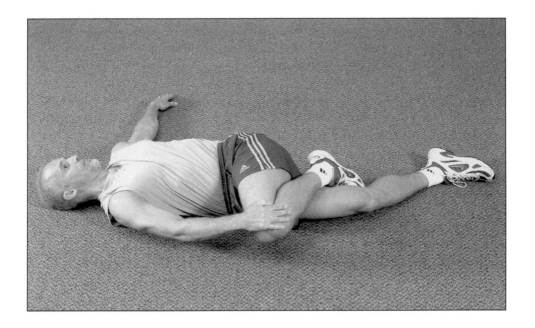

CHEST OUT THEN HUG YOURSELF

Stretches the pecs, shoulders, and upper back

While seated or standing, bring the shoulder blades close together and hold. Then cross the arms across the chest, "hugging" yourself, trying to bring the shoulder blades as far apart as possible, and hold.

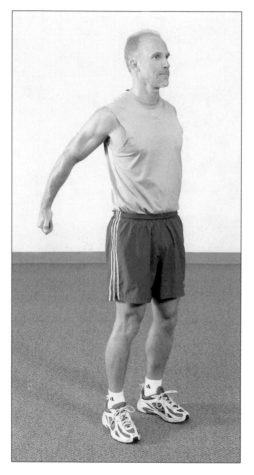 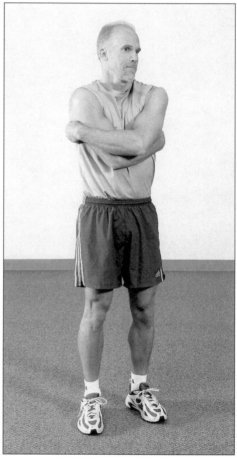

SIX-WAY NECK STRETCH

Stretches the neck muscles

In the seated or standing position, touch the chin to the chest and hold, then tip the head back as far as possible and hold. Next rotate the head to your right as far as possible and hold, then rotate to the left and hold. Next, bend the head, trying to touch the ear to the shoulder, and hold. Repeat on the opposite side.

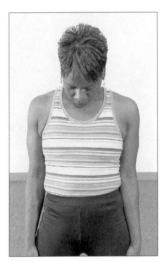 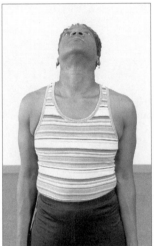 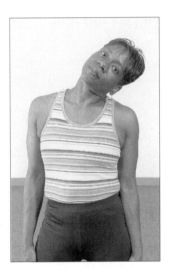

Add the following basic core strength exercises to your flexibility exercises. These can be done daily, in addition to the core exercises described in chapter 5 (pages 106 to 113). These exercises are so easy to do that they should not result in soreness.

SUPERMAN AND X-MAN

Lying facedown with the arms extended overhead, alternate raising the arms as high off the ground as possible. Do the same for your legs. When you get this down, raise one arm and the opposite leg at the same time.

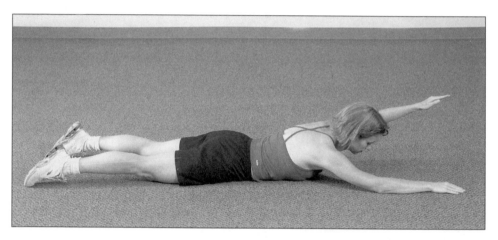

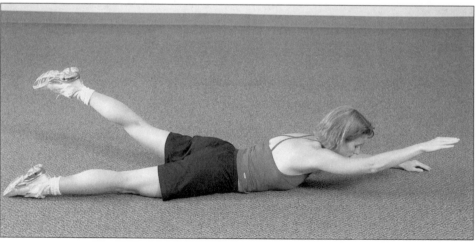

CRUNCH

While lying on your back, place your feet on the ground, cross your arms on your chest, and bend at the hips and knees. Raise your shoulders as high off the floor as possible. For more challenge, do the crunch with your feet on a stool or bench.

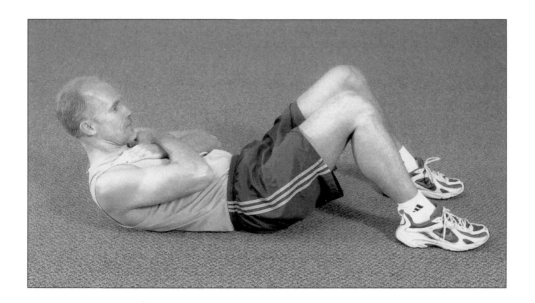

HIP-UP (TRUNK BRIDGE)

While lying on your back with your knees bent, raise your midsection as high off the floor as possible.

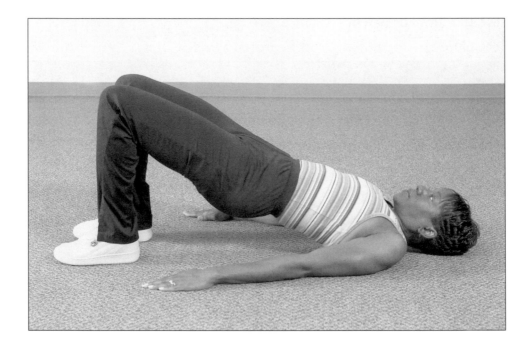

Pilates, Yoga, and Tai Chi

There are several popular forms of exercise that focus on flexibility as a fitness goal. Pilates and yoga are two types of exercise growing rapidly in popularity that emphasize flexibility of all joints, especially the trunk and back. If done properly, both can also be a form of relaxation therapy. Pilates exercise combines flexibility, core strength, calisthenics, and mind–body focus into a moderate-intensity workout. Because of the gracefulness of the movements and the emphasis on mind–body focus, Pilates has been a popular form of training for dancers for quite a while. Yoga has been done in many cultures as a form of active meditation for years. Yoga practices emphasize postures or poses being held for very short periods in order to emphasize flexibility, strength, and mental discipline. Although it sounds difficult, those who regularly practice yoga swear by its relaxing qualities. The different types of yoga can be confusing for the experienced as well as the newbie poser. Experts recommend starting with a beginner's class and deciding if you like the instructor. A good instructor has years of individual yoga practice and experience teaching people of varied skill levels.

Can yoga assist in the control of blood pressure? In a small study of hypertensive patients, roughly 65 percent could control blood pressure with Shavasana yoga only—no drugs needed at all (Sundar et al. 1984). When the patients quit the daily yoga practice, blood pressure rose significantly to prestudy levels. In a more recent small study of persons with hypertension, researchers showed a significant reduction in resting heart rate, systolic pressure, and diastolic pressure after only three weeks of daily yoga

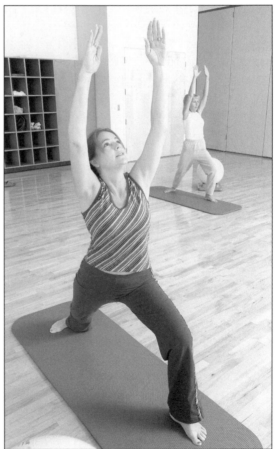

© Human Kinetics

Yoga works well for increasing flexibility and releasing stress, and studies indicate that it helps lower blood pressure, too.

training (Vijayalakshmi et al. 2004). After four weeks of training, there was an even greater reduction in blood pressure and heart rate. Although these are small studies, it appears that the frequent practice of yoga can lower blood pressure.

Other forms of exercise that emphasize overall body flexibility include tai chi, an Asian form of slow controlled movements done in a regular pattern. Teachers emphasize proper form, proper order of movements, and the discipline needed to hold poses (similar to yoga). There is more movement involved in tai chi than yoga, but not much more. Both exercise forms also place a great deal of emphasis on mentally focusing on the present, which also tends to be a great stress reliever. Tai chi is used regularly by those experienced in martial arts because of the similarities between the tai chi movements and several martial arts disciplines.

Preliminary evidence suggests that regular tai chi exercises result in reduced blood pressure and stress. In one study, subjects practiced a 12-week tai chi chuan exercise training program regularly three times per week. Each session included a 10-minute warm-up, 30-minute tai chi exercise, and a 10-minute cool-down. Exercise intensity was estimated to be approximately 64 percent of maximal heart rate. After 12 weeks of tai chi training, the treatment group showed significant decrease in systolic blood pressure of 15.6 mmHg and diastolic blood pressure of 8.8 mmHg (Tsai et al. 2003). Responses to a questionnaire to evaluate tolerance to stress showed that both trait anxiety (a measure of "baseline" or chronic anxiety) and state anxiety (acute anxiety) were decreased in the subjects. In another study, smaller reductions in both systolic and diastolic blood pressure were achieved from a 6-week tai chi program (Lee 2004).

Types of Yoga

Many types and variations of yoga exist. When selecting a yoga class, you may want to know more about the differences in types.

Ashtanga (Astanga): Also known as *power yoga*. The yoga postures flow with an emphasis on strength and agility. This is a very advanced form.

Bikram: A challenging and exhilarating series of postures done in a heated room. This is not recommended if you have poorly controlled blood pressure.

Gentle: Gentle yoga is really a subcategory of classical hatha yoga adapted to the needs of beginners and those with limitations.

Hatha: Forms and traditional postures used most commonly in the U.S. This form is for people of all experience levels.

Iyengar: Emphasizes the precise alignment of a pose. For the experienced, but not advanced.

Kundalini: Kundalini yoga can include chanting, hand positions, breathing techniques, and sometimes a vigorous aerobic-type workout with repetitive motions and little emphasis on form or holding positions. This is a more advanced form.

Moksha: A relatively new form of yoga that combines three forms of yoga: the temperature of hot yoga, the precision of therapeutic yoga, and the foundations of traditional yoga. This advanced form should not be done if blood pressure is not well controlled.

Restorative: Restorative yoga is a subcategory of poses found within other styles, particularly traditional or Iyengar, focusing on poses that are restful and rejuvenating. Restorative yoga is good for beginners.

Viniyoga: This style of yoga practices postures according to an individual's needs and capacities. It is good for beginners, but the instructor's abilities are essential to success.

Summary

The most common reason for not exercising or for giving up an exercise program is the perceived or real lack of available time. If this applies to you, it does not make much sense to focus all of your exercise time on one area, especially flexibility training. Getting flexibility training through a form of regular exercise such as tai chi or martial arts that combines the three basic elements of fitness training is one of the most efficient uses of exercise time when little is available. Personal interests, resources, and availability all will play a role in determining how you spend your exercise time, but consider adding or exploring these types of fitness programs to lend some variety to your plan that will continue to benefit your blood pressure.

ACTION PLAN:
GAINING AND MAINTAINING FLEXIBILITY

☐ Focus on improving flexibility in the problem areas: the lower back, hamstrings, and hip flexors.

☐ Know the difference between ballistic and static stretching.

☐ Learn 10 effective stretches and three core strength exercises that are easy to add to your flexibility routine.

☐ Investigate other options such as yoga, tai chi, and Pilates.

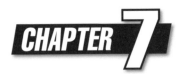
BALANCING HEALTHY EATING, ACTIVITY, AND MEDICATION

A s you know by now, the first step in the management of hypertension is to make the necessary lifestyle adjustments that lower blood pressure. Although the modifications suggested in this book and many other sources are too often ignored by *both* patients and their physicians, these changes can reduce your blood pressure to a range that will keep you off prescribed blood pressure medications. Unfortunately, in the majority of cases, medication is nevertheless needed to manage blood pressure.

How does your physician decide which interventions are best for you to control blood pressure? The decision to prescribe medication, in most cases a medication that will be needed for a lifetime, is not made lightly. In order to assist physicians in their medical management of persons with hypertension, the National Heart, Lung, and Blood Institute in 1997, in the Sixth Report of the Joint National Committee on Prevention, Detection, Evaluation, and Treatment of High Blood Pressure (JNC 6), provided treatment recommendations based on the level of hypertension and the presence of other risk factors. These recommendations were later reinforced and added to in the most recent report, JNC 7, from the same group. In JNC

7, persons with hypertension were stratified by blood pressure "stages" (see also table 1.1 on page 4) as follows:

- Prehypertension: 130–139/85–89
- Stage 1 hypertension: 140–159/90–99
- Stage 2 hypertension: 160–179/100–109

Once the initial level of blood pressure is determined, the physician identifies additional risk factors for heart and vascular disease. As we discussed in chapter 3, your doctor will decide which tests are important for you in order to discern these risk factors. The major risk factors your doctor is looking for include the following:

- Smoking
- Elevated blood cholesterol or triglycerides
- Diabetes
- Family history of cardiovascular diseases

Your physician will also want to assess whether your elevated blood pressure has already resulted in damage to other organs and whether you already have clinical cardiovascular disease. Target organ disease (TOD) includes the following:

- Heart- and coronary-artery–specific disease
  Left ventricular hypertrophy (enlarged heart)
  Angina (heart-related chest pain)
  Prior heart attack
  Prior coronary artery revascularization (either by surgery, angioplasty, or stenting)
  Heart failure
- Previous stroke or transient ischemic attack (TIA)
- Kidney disease
- Peripheral vascular disease
- Retina damage

Lifestyle modifications we have discussed previously and will discuss further in this chapter are recommended for those with prehypertension until a reduction in pressure occurs. Those with stage 1 pressure elevation and no risk factors, disease, or TOD can attempt lifestyle modification strategies without medication for a maximum of 12 months; if that is not successful, a physician will likely recommend medication. Those with stage 1 and at least one risk factor can try lifestyle modification practices for 6 months before considering the addition of medications.

For some, blood pressure medication should begin at the diagnosis of hypertension. Those with stage 2 or higher initial blood pressure, regardless of the presence of risk factors or disease, will need to begin medication and lifestyle modification practices as soon as possible after the diagnosis of hypertension is made. The same is true for those with diabetes or any cardiovascular disease or other TOD—even those with prehypertension will need to begin medication at the diagnosis of hypertension in order to prevent worsening the disease already present. If you have elevated blood pressure and diabetes you will probably need to begin blood pressure medication at a lower blood pressure, in order to achieve a lower blood pressure goal of 130/80 (Chobanian et al. 2003). This lower target will reduce your risk of TOD.

We have focused on the lifestyle modification of exercise and increased physical activity in the previous chapters. In this chapter, we will focus on the importance of other lifestyle modifications, specifically weight loss and healthy eating, both major contributing factors in the battle against hypertension. The basic nutrients and principles of dietary planning are explained, especially as they relate to management of blood pressure. We'll also discuss the six common classes of medications prescribed for high blood pressure and how these medications work if you're exercising and eating right.

Principles of Healthy Eating and Weight Loss

Weight loss is a top goal for many people, and for good reason. Maintaining a healthy weight helps lower blood pressure, along with the risk for certain diseases and other health problems. In fact, weight loss can reduce blood pressure independent of adding regular exercise. If you lose weight you can expect a 5 to 20 mmHg reduction per 10 kilograms of body weight lost along the way down to an ideal BMI (see calculation in chapter 3) between 18.5 to 24.9 (Chobanian et al. 2003). Of course, the only way most people could expect to lose this much weight is to reduce caloric intake and adopt a program of regular exercise as described in this book. Once the weight is off, it is absolutely essential to maintain your body weight and BMI in the ideal 18.5 to 24.9 range, to continue to keep your blood pressure in the ideal range.

Purposeful healthy eating with a goal of losing weight can lead to great accomplishment. It takes planning, though, and an understanding of some basic numbers and calculations. Let's start with the concept of *energy balance*. In essence, this principle means that if the energy you put into your body (in the form of calories through food and fluids) equals the energy you put out (through your basal metabolic rate, physical activity, exercise, and digestion), you are in energy balance and your weight is maintained. To lose weight, the amount of calories you expend should be higher than the amount you take in. The *basal metabolic rate (BMR)* is the amount of energy to keep "all systems go"—that is, the amount required for all your body's involuntary activities, such as keeping your heart beating, opening and closing blood vessels, maintaining breathing, digesting food, and fueling your brain and nerves. The caloric energy used with BMR helps to fuel the internal heater that maintains body temperature. BMR is what people think they are referring to when they describe themselves as having slow or fast "metabolism." Many diets have promised to generate a higher BMR if one eats foods creating a greater "thermic effect"—that is, these diets encourage you to eat foods that require a greater amount of energy to metabolize than they provide in caloric intake. There are a few foods like that; most have an extremely high water content and are very low in calories. In reality, it is important to remember that even under the best circumstances BMR accounts for only about 10 percent (in most cases under 10 percent) of the body's daily energy demands. Because this value is usually so low, for our purposes, we will not include the thermal effect in further discussions of BMR.

The best way to increase your BMR contribution toward your daily caloric expenditure is to exercise. Individuals with a greater amount of lean body mass (mostly muscle weight) have a higher BMR than those

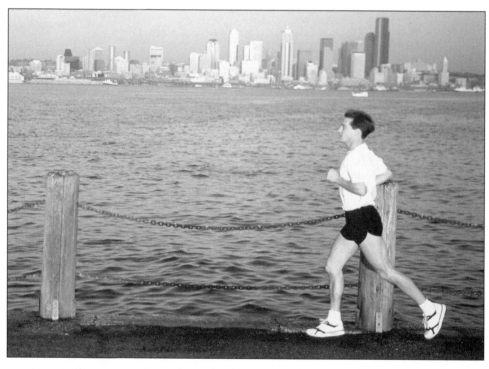

© Photodisc

Activities that require high energy expenditure, such as running, are quite effective for weight loss and can also help increase your basal metabolic rate.

with less lean body weight. As you might expect, BMR is influenced by regular exercise training. People who are fit have more lean weight and thus a higher BMR.

The following sidebar contains some of the numbers and concepts that we just talked about, along with some other essential information. Some of these items are explained in more detail in the following sections. Feel free to come back to this list later as a quick reference to the facts.

Important Numbers for Weight Loss

- ▸ For every pound lost, expect a decrease in blood pressure of about 1 percent
- ▸ Calories in = calories from food + fluids + supplements
- ▸ Calories out = basal metabolic rate (BMR) + activity + exercise
- ▸ Thermic effect = usually 10 percent of caloric intake
- ▸ 1 pound fat = 3,500 calories
- ▸ 1 pound protein or carbohydrate = 2,000 calories
- ▸ Stored glycogen as fuel source: 2,000 calories per pound
- ▸ Water weight 4:1 or 4 pounds water to 1 pound glycogen
- ▸ Daily physical activity—usually an additional 20 percent of BMR
- ▸ Exercise: Ideally should be 250 to 300 calories per day

Fat

The cardinal rule of weight loss is to consume fewer calories than you expend, so of course it is essential to limit the foods that are the densest in calories. Fat is the most calorie-dense type of food at about 9 calories per gram, or 3,500 calories per pound. Carbohydrate and protein, at 4 calories per gram, are less than half the calorie density of fat. Excess fat in the diet is associated with increased risk of coronary artery disease, vascular disease, stroke, and high blood pressure. Most of us need to eat less fat.

Unfortunately, these rich foods typically taste pretty good, and most of us find a lot of satisfaction in rich, good-tasting, filling foods. Put a piece of calorie-dense cheesecake (900 calories per slice) and a piece of celery (30 calories) in front of 10 people, and one oddball might pick the celery but the rest of us are going to scarf up every last crumb of the cheesecake. Add a little peanut butter (100 calories), cream cheese (200 calories), or blue cheese (300 calories) to the celery and a few more of us are going to opt for the good food as opposed to the feel-good food. The trick is not to eliminate all the fat and calories but to reduce them to a level that helps us achieve and maintain a healthy weight.

Low fat also equals lower risk for heart disease. A diet lower in fat typically lowers serum cholesterol and triglycerides, both of which contribute to plaque development in the arteries. When it comes to fat, however, not all types are equal. In fact, there are the good (unsaturated) fats, the bad (saturated) fats, and the ugly (trans, or processed) fats.

The good fats.   Fats from plants, such as corn oil, olive oil, and canola oil, are less likely to cause artery-clogging plaque buildup. A good way to identify a good fat is to observe its state at room temperature. Generally, unsaturated fats are liquid, whereas saturated fats, which have higher melting points, are solid. Omega-3 fats, found primarily in fish oils, have antioxidant effects that are beneficial in reducing the risks of developing or worsening many diseases, including hypertension.

The bad fats.   Saturated fats are high in calories and high in cholesterol. Sources of saturated fat include animal products (meats and cheeses), coconut, and coconut oil. Saturated fats are usually solid or almost solid at room temperature. Once absorbed into the bloodstream, saturated fats contribute to the buildup of plaque along the inside walls of arteries, resulting in elevated blood pressure and end-organ damage, especially heart attacks and strokes.

The ugly fats.   Touted for years as an acceptable diet alternative, trans fats are used extensively in prepared baked goods, crackers, and other seemingly harmless "low-fat" items. Recent research has found that not only does trans fat add to the caloric intake and cholesterol level, but it also robs the body of beneficial high-density cholesterol (HDL). Try to avoid trans fats.

Carbohydrate

With the recent "low-carb" craze, carbohydrate has come to occupy a prominent place in the public consciousness. But do most people really know what a carbohydrate is? The simplest explanation is that a carbohydrate is a sugar molecule. It is necessary for energy production, especially for the brain, which can use only carbohydrate for fuel. Too much carbohydrate in our diet can result in the development of diabetes and vascular disease. Experts tell us that the bulk of the calories in our diet, roughly 50 to 60 percent of our daily caloric intake, should come from carbohydrate, ideally complex carbohydrate.

There are many forms of carbohydrate, divided primarily into simple, smaller molecules such as table sugar and milk and fruit sugar and complex carbohydrate, mainly vegetable fiber and starches. The body uses these two types of carbohydrate in different fashions. Simple carbohydrate is quickly digested, absorbed into the bloodstream, and taken up by active tissues with the help of the hormone insulin (which increases with the elevation of simple sugar in the bloodstream). Complex carbohydrate, by virtue of its increased molecular size, takes longer to digest and become absorbed. The slower rate of absorption results in less insulin release, yet complex carbohydrate is still readily available to working tissues.

Extra insulin causes a cascade of events resulting in insulin resistance, or type 2 diabetes (also called adult-onset diabetes). First, excess insulin initially results in an increase in carbohydrate utilization, which dramatically lowers the blood sugar levels, creating (among other things) increased hunger. This is one of our cues to eat again. If our diet consists of simple sugar, we tend to eat more because we burn more. Over time this repeated release of insulin results in our tissues becoming trained to take up and burn carbohydrate only when the insulin is at a higher level. The body requires more and more insulin to utilize the carbohydrate. Eventually the body is unable to produce enough insulin to "turn on" the tissue gate to the carbohydrate in the bloodstream, and the blood sugar, or glucose level, becomes chronically elevated. This increase in the body's insulin resistance is referred to as *type 2 diabetes,* and it is a health problem on the rise in both the adult and adolescent populations.

Low-Carbohydrate Diets

For years the late Dr. Robert Atkins promoted a diet rich in protein and low in insulin-producing, storage-inducing carbohydrate. Initially popular in the 1970s, Dr. Atkins' plan has seen a dramatic resurgence in popularity and staying power since the late 1990s, more so than any previous fad diets. Books touting low-carbohydrate plans are regularly on the best-seller lists. Low-carbohydrate versions of normally high-carbohydrate products such as breads and cereals are available. There is even a "low-carb" peanut butter (peanut butter normally is low in carbohydrate). Restaurants seem to be adding and promoting their low-carbohydrate items everywhere. Why is this?

In a phrase, it works. Yes, you more than likely will lose weight, feel better, and perhaps even reduce your cardiac risk factors while on the diet. But at what cost? (That is, aside from the $3 you shell out for a loaf of low-carbohydrate bread.) Anyone who has suffered through the first few weeks of a low-carbohydrate diet will describe it as a living hell. At first, dramatically reducing your carbohydrate intake to 20 to 100 grams per day is not too bad. But that craving for a single slice of lifeless white bread gets stronger as the week goes on and your body continues to burn up the stored carbohydrate (glycogen) in the muscles and liver. After this has burned off (about 100 grams on average) your body goes after the stored fat: Remember, *the brain functions only on the high-octane carbohydrate energy source* and will dictate that your body pump sugar to the needy brain cells at any cost. So, the body goes into fat breakdown, or *ketosis.* The blood sugar supply goes up to the brain, but so do the by-products:

nasty ketones. Ketones in excess make you feel horrible. This is when most of the low-carbohydrate dropouts occur. Fatigue and irritability are the hallmarks of this stage.

Do the math: As the body rids itself of stored glycogen without replenishing the store from glucose in the diet, will weight loss occur? A normal amount of stored glycogen is about 500 grams (1 pound), or about 2,000 calories of energy. This is generally enough for one or two days' worth of potential energy for the average inactive person. As the glycogen is depleted, water is also lost. For every gram of glycogen, 4 grams of water is lost. So once the glycogen is completely gone, about 5 pounds is lost. Any carbohydrate consumed that is not immediately used will then be restored in muscle along with four times the amount of water. The initial 5 pounds of weight loss is at best temporary for most people. A portion of fluid weight is gained back as the body strives to maintain normal hydration. Additionally, to continue the normal requirements for blood sugar throughout the body—specifically the brain—fat is broken down and used. It takes motivation to stay with this type of diet. Once you begin eating carbohydrate again, the weight you lost will return. Other potential health problems with a low-carbohydrate diet include elevated cholesterol levels, gout (excess protein by-products in the blood that lodge in the joints, creating a very painful arthritis), and kidney disease.

The Low Glycemic Index Diet

As you now know, carbohydrate has traditionally been divided into simple (sweet foods causing large and rapid changes in blood sugar levels) and complex (more fiber-containing foods that produce a sustained, slower change in blood sugar levels). This is the basis for a useful way to define carbohydrate foods, which is known as the glycemic index (GI). The GI is a ranking of foods from 0 to 100 based on the blood sugar response after ingestion compared to a reference food, either glucose or white bread. A higher GI indicates that a food is ideal for rapid energy *availability* and a lower GI promotes energy *restoration.* The body's response to food is affected by several factors, including age, activity level, insulin level, time of day, amount of fiber and fat in the food, how refined (processed) the food is, and what was eaten with the food. In addition to these, other factors such as the ratio of carbohydrate to fat and protein, as well as how the food was cooked (for example, boiled compared to fried or baked), and metabolism will determine the way your body's sugar level responds after eating.

Processed pasta, white bread, and certain varieties of potatoes are usually high on the glycemic index. Other high-GI foods are most varieties of white rice, soft drinks, ice cream, chocolate bars, and candy. Because of a higher grain and fiber content and less processing, whole-grain or rye breads and pastas are lower on the glycemic index. Other examples of low-GI foods are wheat bran, barley cereals, oats, fruit, lentils, soybeans, and baked beans. Table 7.1 shows more GI rankings for various foods.

Table 7.1 Glycemic Index Values for Common Foods

The following list shows the food category and the glycemic index for each particular food in that category.

Food category	Food	Glycemic index
Breads	White bread	70
	Whole grain bread	69
	Pumpernickel	41
	Dark rye	76
	Sourdough	57
	Heavy mixed grain	30–45
Legumes	Lentils	28
	Soybeans	18
	Baked beans (canned)	48
Breakfast cereals	Cornflakes	84
	Rice Bubbles	82
	Cheerios	83
	Puffed Wheat	80
	All-Bran	42
	Porridge	46
Snack foods	Mars bar	65
	Jelly beans	80
	Chocolate bar	49
Fruits	Apple	38
	Orange	44
	Peach	42
	Banana	55
	Watermelon	72
Dairy foods	Milk, whole	27
	Milk, skim	32
	Ice cream, full fat	61
	Yogurt, low fat, with fruit	33
Soft drinks and sports drinks	Fanta	68
	Gatorade	78

Reprinted from www.glycemicindex.com, by permission of Professor J. Brand-Miller.

Low-GI food is especially helpful in assisting those who want to lose weight. As a result of a slower digestion time, low glycemic index foods will increase the sugar levels in the body to sustain energy levels for longer periods. This means the appetite is usually decreased because energy is being slowly released into the bloodstream. On the other hand, faster-metabolized carbohydrate that has a high glycemic index is great for raising low blood sugar after intense exercise. Health experts encourage using the glycemic index in conjunction with other meal programs to assist in managing diabetes and controlling weight.

In the big "diet picture" we must look at the total of what we eat, not just individual foods. Also, regardless of the type of diet, portion control is the foundation for success. In order to look at the big picture we need to look at the daily *glycemic load.* One unit of glycemic load (GL) is equal to the glycemic effect of 1 gram of glucose. Glycemic load is equal to the glycemic index (GI) times the grams of carbohydrate per serving. A typical diet has about 100 glycemic load units per day, though it can range from 60 to 180. An important point to keep in mind is that the glycemic load is not the type of carbohydrate consumed, but the amount.

The Low-GI Way to Lose Weight

- ▶ Eat breakfast cereals made with oats, barley, and bran.
- ▶ Eat "grainy" breads made with whole seeds.
- ▶ Reduce the amount of potatoes you eat.
- ▶ Reduce the amount of *everything* you eat.
- ▶ Enjoy all types of fruit and vegetables (but limit potatoes).
- ▶ Eat plenty of salads consisting of vegetables with vinaigrette dressing.

Protein

The third major nutrient in our diet is protein. Protein provides the essential building blocks for all of the body's tissues, is the major oxygen-carrying component of blood (hemoglobin), and is the main biochemical component of many of the body's essential enzymes and hormones. We need protein to grow as well as to maintain all essential body structures and functions. Probably because of its essential role in these functions, protein is the least-used form of caloric energy. The body will preferentially break down and use carbohydrate and fat before breaking down protein to make energy. In addition to the loss of lean tissue weight (remember the discussion on BMR), when the body uses protein for fuel it creates several by-products, mainly ketones. This substance is what drives more people off low-carbohydrate diets than anything else because elevated ketones make you feel bad.

It is important to maintain a regular intake of protein in the diet. Unfortunately, some high-protein foods are also high in fats, particular artery-clogging saturated fats. Generally vegetables, nuts, and grains have less fat and should make up the bulk of your protein intake if you have hypertension or any of the other diseases associated with hypertension.

A special note: Those who have extremely high blood pressure (greater than 200/110) and those who have kidney disease as a result of hypertension may need to limit the amount of protein in the diet. If your kidney function has slowed because of disease, your doctor may recommend a lower-protein diet. This is something very important to discuss with your doctor in order to reduce the risk of complications due to kidney failure.

Sodium

In most people, sodium acts as a strong magnet for fluid, causing fluid retention. More fluid results in higher pressure in the blood vessels and, obviously, higher blood pressure. In African-Americans and Hispanics, the fluid magnet effect of dietary sodium is even stronger. In Anglos and Asians, the sodium magnet effect is less.

Obviously, in those who are more "salt sensitive," monitoring the amount of dietary sodium is an essential component in the medical management of high blood pressure. Recent research findings indicate that those with high blood pressure should consume less than 2 grams of dietary sodium per day. This can lower your blood pressure 2 to 8 mmHg (Chobanian et al. 2003).

For some, restricting sodium constitutes a dramatic change in dietary habits. Eliminating salt, bacon, lunch meat, canned soups, and chips can be a major ordeal if those items are staples in your diet. Trying a variety of foods is one way to broaden your tastes to include low-sodium items in your diet. Experimenting with different spice combinations and the use of salt substitutes has helped many in their quest to reduce sodium. It takes about three weeks for a change in routine to become habit, or to be accepted without much thought into our routine. Getting used to a dietary taste, be it low sodium, low fat, or low carbohydrate, takes about that long.

Avoiding the Pitfalls of Eating Out

In 2000, the average American dined outside the home 4.2 times per week. If the food selection at restaurants consisted mostly of fruits and vegetables, and the portions were appropriate for an individual rather than a family of four, then eating outside the home would not be too bad. Unfortunately, menu selections are generally higher in fat, processed carbohydrate, and sodium than home-cooked food is, and portions are bigger because we want to receive the most for our money. Restaurant owners are generally smart people and know we will be less likely to come back to their establishment if we walk away from a paid-for meal less than pleasantly stuffed. The result: The more often you eat outside the home, the more likely it is that you will have a few extra pounds hanging around your midsection.

So if you dine out often, what should you do to maintain your health? First, overcome the concept that the best value for your money means a large quantity of food rather than high quality food. Never, never "super-size" your meal or eat anything more than a child's portion of fast food. A meal consisting of a "supersized" cheeseburger, fries, and nondiet soft drink packs 1,825 calories: Check your BMRs (basal metabolic rates) and caloric expenditure for ADLs (activities for daily living) and not many of you will find much more room for anything else to eat that day. For some of you, this one meal will exceed your caloric requirement for an entire day. Not bad for economic caloric value: about 0.27 cents per calorie!

Skip appetizers, which are notoriously unhealthy—worse than most desserts for fat content. For example, the caloric content of a deep-fried onion or cheese-based dip will exceed that of the entrée and dessert *combined*. A noncream soup works well as a starter. Speaking of dessert, try not to do that either, unless it's fresh fruit.

Restaurant Items to Avoid

When dining out, try to steer clear of the following:

- Pastries
- Fried anything
- Crispy anything
- Breaded anything
- Creamed anything
- Foods described as buttery or au gratin
- Buffets
- All-you-can eat specials
- Happy hour specials
- Alfredo sauces
- Gravy
- Coconut milk, palm oil

With all these don'ts, you may wonder what's left. In just about any restaurant, you can find entrée items that are steamed, broiled, grilled, charbroiled, poached, or fresh. Portion control is key. Order a lunch portion when possible. The ideal meat portion is 3 ounces, about the size of a deck of cards. If you get a larger cut of meat, take the rest home for another meal. Order one entrée and split it with your dining companion. Order your favorite vegetables. Fill your tank with a couple of glasses of water—without any additional spirits—before the meal arrives. A light beer (around 100 calories) before dinner will also help to fill you up more quickly.

The DASH Diet

The Dietary Approaches to Stop Hypertension diet, commonly known as the DASH diet, is one of the most well-researched diet plans to help control blood pressure. This plan helps decrease the risk of many diseases by incorporating healthy eating habits into one's lifestyle. Used in combination with an exercise program, this diet can help you lose weight. Of 459 middle-aged adults (average age 44 years) tested, over half (59 percent) were African-American and 49 percent were women. The average prediet blood pressure was 132/85. Participants were assigned to follow either their normal diet (control diet), a diet rich in fruits and vegetables (fruit and vegetable diet), or a diet that was not only rich in fruits and vegetables but was also rich in low-fat dairy products and low in saturated fat (combination diet). They followed the diets for 11 weeks.

The combination diet significantly lowered both systolic and diastolic blood pressure, while the fruit and vegetable diet lowered only systolic blood pressure. The most important observation was that the group who reduced their total saturated fat intake with a diet rich in fruits, vegetables, and low-fat dairy foods significantly lowered blood pressure—as much as an antihypertensive medication would. The effects of the diets on blood pressure were evident within one week, reaching maximum benefit after two weeks. Those with higher baseline blood pressure received the greatest effect of the diet on lowering blood pressure. Both men and women had comparable decreases in blood pressure (Appel et al. 1997). In the bigger picture, a blood pressure decrease of the magnitude seen in the DASH diet is estimated to reduce the incidence of coronary artery disease by 15 percent and stroke by 27 percent. See diet details in table 7.2.

A second diet study called "DASH-Sodium" compared the blood-pressure–lowering effects of the DASH diet and levels of daily sodium intake. The group consuming the lowest amount of daily sodium, 1,500 mg, had the greatest reduction in blood pressure (Sacks et al. 2001). Convenience or processed foods and snacks typically have a high sodium and salt content. These include canned vegetables, condiments, and soups. Cured meats, such as bacon, jerky, and ham, also contain high amounts of sodium. To reduce your daily sodium, don't add salt in the cooking process or at the table. Choose low- or no-sodium canned and processed foods. Avoid highly salted snack foods and nuts.

Table 7.2 The DASH Diet

Food group	Daily servings	Serving sizes	Examples and notes	Significance to the DASH eating plan
Grains and grain products	7–8	1 slice bread; 1 oz dry cereal*; 1/2 cup cooked cereals, rice, or pasta	Whole-wheat bread, English muffin, pita bread, bagel, cereals, grits, oatmeal, crackers, unsalted pretzels, popcorn	Major sources of energy and fiber
Vegetables	4–5	1 cup raw leafy vegetables, 1/2 cup cooked vegetables, 6 oz (150 ml) vegetable juice	Tomatoes, potatoes, carrots, peas, squash, broccoli, turnip greens, collards, kale, spinach, artichokes, green beans, lima beans, sweet potatoes	Rich sources of potassium, magnesium, and fiber
Fruits	4–5	1 medium fruit; 1/4 cup dried fruit; 1/2 cup fresh, frozen, or canned fruit; 6 oz (150 ml) fruit juice	Apricots, bananas, dates, grapes, oranges, orange juice, grapefruit, mangoes, melons, peaches, pineapples, prunes, raisins, strawberries, tangerines	Important sources of potassium, magnesium, and fiber
Low-fat or nonfat dairy foods	2–3	8 oz (200 ml) milk, 1 cup yogurt, 1.5 oz (40 g) cheese	Skim or semiskim milk, nonfat or low-fat frozen yogurt, nonfat or low-fat cheese	Major sources of calcium and protein

Food group	Daily servings	Serving sizes	Examples and notes	Significance to the DASH eating plan
Meats, poultry, and fish	2 or less	3 oz (80 g) cooked meat, poultry, or fish	Lean cuts with visible fat trimmed away; broiled, roasted, boiled instead of fried; skin removed from poultry	Rich sources of protein and magnesium
Nuts, seeds, and dry beans	4–5 per week	1.5 oz or 1/3 cup nuts, 2 tbsp or .5 oz seeds, 1/2 cup cooked dry beans	Almonds, mixed nuts, peanuts, sunflower seeds, kidney beans, lentils	Rich sources of energy, magnesium, potassium, protein, and fiber
Fats and oils**	2–3	1 tsp soft margarine, 1 tbsp low-fat mayonnaise, 2 tbsp light salad dressing, 1 tsp vegetable oil	Soft margarine, low-fat mayonnaise, light salad dressing, vegetable oil (such as olive, corn, canola, or safflower)	DASH has 27 percent of calories as fat, including fat in or added to foods
Sweets	5	1 tbsp sugar, 1 tbsp jelly or jam, .5 oz jelly beans, 8 oz lemonade	Maple syrup, sugar, jelly, jam, fruit-flavored gelatin, jelly beans, hard candy, fruit punch, sorbet, ices	Sweets should be low in fat

*Equals 1/2 to 1 1/4 cups, depending on cereal type. Check the product's Nutrition Facts Label.

**Fat content changes serving counts for fats and oils: For example, 1 tbsp of regular salad dressing equals 1 serving; 1 tbsp of a low-fat dressing equals 1/2 serving; 1 tbsp of a nonfat dressing equals 0 servings.

From the National Heart, Lung and Blood Institute and the National Institutes of Health (NIH), a section of the US Department of Health and Human Services. www.nhlbi.nih.gov/health/public/heart/hbp/dash/new_dash.pdf

Further Information on DASH

For an excellent information source on the DASH diet from food selection to meal planning, point your Web browser to the following link: www.nhlbi.nih.gov/health/public/heart/hbp/dash/new_dash.pdf

The DASH diet is a healthy alternative for reducing blood pressure and helps you with your weight-loss goals. More important, the DASH diet is a sensible diet that you can realistically follow for the rest of your life. To begin the diet, simply make your mealtime selections based on the information in table 7.2. Make sure you follow the portion guidelines—no cheating! Try to spread your meals throughout the day and eat at least the minimum amount of fruits and vegetables.

Choosing Medication for an Active Lifestyle

Currently it is estimated that up to 50 percent of those with hypertension are either undermedicated or not medicated at all in order to reduce blood pressure to an appropriate level. Drug therapy can reduce mortality from causes related to high blood pressure by as much as 21 percent. For those who exercise regularly as a lifestyle modification to control blood pressure, choosing a medication that does not affect exercise ability can be a challenge.

The six classes of blood pressure medications found to improve overall outcomes are

- diuretics (primarily thiazides),
- ACE inhibitors,
- angiotensin II receptor blockers (ARBs),
- beta-blockers,
- alpha-blockers, and
- long-acting calcium channel receptor blockers.

Other classes of antihypertensive agents may be added to the six basic classes if blood pressure is not adequately controlled with a single drug and lifestyle changes. JNC 7 advises physicians to add a second drug when a combination of lifestyle changes and the initial drug does not reduce blood pressure to the target range or if the initial elevated pressure is 20/10 mmHg above the target range (Chobanian et al. 2003). In fact, more than 60 percent of patients in all major medication research trials have required two or more antihypertensive medications in order to reach ideal blood pressure. Table 7.3 lists generic and brand names of drugs in the six classes, along with common side effects.

Table 7.3 Classes of Common Hypertension Medications

Class	Selected examples Generic name (Product name)	Side effects
ACE inhibitors	Captopril (Capoten), enalapril (Vasotec), lisinopril (Prinivil, Zestril), ramipril (Altace)	Cough, low potassium, rash
Alpha-blockers	Doxazosin (Cardura), prazosin (Minipress), terazosin (Hytrin)	Sudden drop in blood pressure when standing, significant elevation of blood pressure with a missed dose
ARB antagonists	Irbesatan (Avapro), losartan (Cozaar), valsatan (Diovan)	Low potassium
Beta-blockers	Atenolol (Tenormin), bisoprolol (Ziabeta), metaprolol (Lopressor, Toprol XL), propranolol (Inderal)	Aggravated asthma, low heart rate, masked symptoms of low blood sugar
Calcium channel receptor blockers	Amlodipine (Norvasc), nifedipine (Adalat, Procardia), diltiazem (Cardizem, Tiazac), verapamil (Calan, Covera-HS, Isoptin-SR, Verelan)	Constipation, low heart rate, swelling of the legs
Diuretics	Hydrochlorothiazide (Esidrix, Ezide, Hydro-par, Oretic), furosemide (Lasix), torsemide (Demadex)	Low potassium, elevated blood sugar

Thiazide diuretics.   In terms of cost, blood pressure control, and low overall side effect rates, thiazides are the first choice of many physicians for their newly diagnosed hypertensive patients. In the latest JNC 7 recommendations, thiazides are recommended for most new persons with stage 1 hypertension. Diuretics have an additive, or *synergistic,* effect with all other classes of antihypertensive drugs. In other words, if your first blood pressure control drug was not a thiazide diuretic, the second one should be. In exercising individuals, however, thiazides can lower potassium and fluid levels. Because of these potential adverse effects in exercisers, sports physicians generally shy away from thiazides as the first choice for active individuals, especially those living in hot climates. Also on the downside, thiazide treatment may increase serum uric acid, resulting in symptoms of gout; have small adverse effects on insulin resistance; and increase lipid levels. Despite these common side effects, long-term studies have shown repeatedly that thiazides are one of the safest and most effective blood pressure medications.

ACE inhibitors.   A solid choice for an initial medication for active individuals, ACE inhibitors are effective at reducing blood pressure and have beneficial effects on other diseases. The use of ACE inhibitors by individuals with diabetic kidney disease and congestive heart disease has become common practice. This class of drugs has very few side effects, the most common being a dry cough. Another less common but more serious side effect is *angioedema,* or a severe allergic reaction involving the respiratory system. There is a rare group of people who have *exercise-induced allergic symptoms.* For this reason, most doctors avoid this drug class in treating people who have a history of severe allergic reactions. Individuals who have multiple allergies who begin taking an ACE inhibitor should be closely monitored during the initial stages of taking the medication.

ARBs.   Angiotensin II receptor blockers (ARBs) are the newest class of drugs for the treatment of hypertension. They are similar to ACE inhibitors in terms of their effectiveness and action, but some important differences exist. First, pharmacologically, the drug's action is at a more specific angiotensin II receptor instead of at a larger number of multiple angiotensin receptors. Dry cough is not a common side effect, and the occurrence or worsening of angioedema is less common than with ACE inhibitors. The number of long-term studies comparing this drug to others is, understandably, few at present. Like other new medications, this class of medications is expensive, and generic versions are not yet available. However, because of their overall effectiveness in reducing blood pressure with few side effects, these drugs appear to be the best first-choice medication for many active individuals.

Beta-blockers.   This well-researched group of medications has been on the market for many years. Beta-blockers work primarily by blocking the effects of catecholamines (adrenaline and stress-induced chemical messengers) on target organs such as the heart and blood vessels. Within the beta-blocker class are selective blockers, which block receptors primarily at the heart, and nonselective blockers, which block beta-receptors everywhere in the body. Because beta-blockers reduce the metabolic demands of the heart muscle by slowing the heart rate and reducing the force of the contraction, they have been shown to increase longevity in patients with coronary artery disease who have had a heart attack. Beta-blockers have been shown to reduce the recurrence of congestive heart failure symptoms and stroke in patients with hypertension. These drugs may also have benefits for patients with other health problems, such as migraine headaches, hyperthyroidism, and anxiety. Side effects of beta-blockers include the masking of symptoms of low blood sugar (hypoglycemia) in people with diabetes who take insulin, as well as possible worsening of asthma symptoms in persons with lung disease.

As with most prescription drugs, this class of drug in particular should be used cautiously and never stopped without the direct supervision and advice of a physician. Very active individuals may find that they cannot achieve the same level of exercise performance while using beta-blockers. Because beta-blockers lower resting and exercising heart rate, maximum and near-maximum exercise ability can be adversely effected. Beta-blocker use can also alter heat-regulating abilities, so people working out in warm climates should use them with caution. For these reasons, most active individuals with hypertension, unless they have one of the aforementioned conditions that benefit from the use of beta-blocking therapy, should try another drug or combination of drugs before beginning beta-blocker therapy.

Alpha-blockers. These drugs, such as clonidine and methyldopa, affect blood pressure by blocking catecholamine effects on the alpha smooth muscle receptors surrounding blood vessels, resulting in less resistance to blood flow. There are very few side effects of this class of drug and no specific side effects for exercisers. Alpha-blockers are a good choice for exercisers who are very good at taking medications daily and not missing or forgetting a dose. The most serious potential side effect is *rebound hypertension,* or a sudden increase in blood pressure, if a dose of the medication is missed. Alpha-blockers must be taken on a regular basis—one single missed dose can cause a dramatic increase in blood pressure resulting in a *hypertensive crisis* (pressures in excess of 200/110 mmHg), which in turn can cause permanent end-organ damage such as heart attack, strokes, or kidney failure. For this reason, the pressure should be reduced and closely monitored in the emergency department or during an inpatient hospital stay.

Calcium-channel receptor blockers. As a group, CRBs control blood pressure by acting to relax the smooth muscle lining of blood vessels. A few specific types of CRBs can also slow heart rate, similar to the heart-rate–controlling effects of beta-blockers. Also similar to beta-blockers, CRBs may decrease maximum and near-maximum exercise performance. Users also report increased fluid retention and constipation as common side effects.

When Medication Is Necessary

Ray is a 35-year-old fireman who was not having any symptoms of blood pressure problems. During a routine annual physical, it was discovered that his blood pressure was elevated to 150/100. He was not overweight, did not smoke, was active both on the job and recreationally, and followed a fairly healthy diet. His only fault was picking two individuals as parents who also developed high blood pressure in their 30s.

With few lifestyle modification options available, Ray's physician decided to start him on medication on his second visit with an elevated pressure. Because of his occupational demands and recreational activities (running, weightlifting, and softball), his physician prescribed an ARB as the initial blood pressure–control drug. On his first follow-up visit, Ray's pressure was down to 136/88, not quite the ideal of less than 120/80, so it was decided to increase the once-daily dosage. Three weeks later, his pressure had dropped to 118/74, and Ray was experiencing no side effects. Despite the early victory, Ray sadly wondered, "Will I be on this medication for the rest of my life?" Without any known reversible cause and an already healthy lifestyle, it looked like the answer was probably yes. In the two years since he began the medication, he has continued to do very well and has come to accept his daily need for medication.

Summary

Lifestyle modifications and medication are necessary for many to manage blood pressure. Think for a minute about the spinoff effects that regular exercise has on lowering blood pressure: If you follow the exercise plans in this book you will lose weight. If you exercise and lose weight, you will lower your blood pressure. If you follow the DASH diet you will consume fewer calories and less sodium and alcohol, and you'll probably lower your blood pressure even more. And it goes without saying that most people who are good exercisers don't smoke.

So at this point you have all the evidence. If you had to make one lifestyle modification, one important change in your life, in order to take control of your blood pressure, what would it be?

BALANCING HEALTHY EATING, ACTIVITY, AND MEDICATION

- ☐ Talk to your doctor about whether your hypertension level allows you to try lifestyle modifications before resorting to medication.

- ☐ Practice the concept of energy balance in your life: energy in = energy out.

- ☐ Reduce fat and sodium in your diet, while incorporating appropriate amounts of carbohydrate and protein.

- ☐ Try the DASH diet by following the guidelines in table 7.2.

- ☐ Be familiar with the types of medication used for lowering blood pressure, and discuss with your doctor any concerns you have about side effects or the drugs' interactions with exercise.

CHAPTER 8

MONITORING PROGRESS AND SPURRING IMPROVEMENT

A dherence to exercise and health programs is an art as well as a science. We know the benefits of exercise, healthy eating, and taking medication, but if we don't follow the plan, we won't get those benefits. We've discussed the most important steps in controlling blood pressure:

1. Exercise regularly and become more physically active.
2. Achieve and maintain a desirable body weight.
3. Adopt healthy eating habits by choosing smaller portions and foods lower in sodium and fat.
4. Take blood pressure medication if it has been prescribed.

In this chapter we'll focus on ways to ensure your success at following these steps: motivating yourself, avoiding common barriers to an exercise program, and adjusting your plan when needed. We'll also talk about how to know when you are ready to go to the next level in a fitness program and the basics of blood pressure monitoring.

How You Can Best "Stick to It"

▸ Identify support mechanisms: people, places, and things.

▸ Avoid overuse injury.

▸ Maintain time flexibility and creativity.

• Traveling

• Weather changes

• Time

• Location

▸ Anticipate roadblocks and be proactive with a plan in writing.

▸ Make a written contract with yourself or others.

▸ Set realistic goals and make a timely plan to achieve them.

▸ Do something you like.

Getting and Staying Motivated

Even though you know the many benefits of exercise and healthy eating, it can still be a challenge to get yourself excited about following through with your well-laid plans. Even avid exercisers are well acquainted with the feeling of just not *wanting* to go out for a run or hop on the bike. There are other motivation squelchers, such as lack of support from others, not having enough time, getting stopped by barriers, boredom with a program, and injury. The key is to find ways around these obstacles. Have a plan for each of these situations so that you can make the most of your program.

Depend on Your Support Staff

It has been well known for years that the success or failure of any significant lifestyle change is directly related to the level of support from those of influence surrounding you. Usually these are the people you live with, but your support group can certainly extend to those in your work or social circles. The new exerciser is more likely to be successful in obtaining fitness goals with a supportive spouse. How do we define a supportive spouse? Well, the cheerleader type works for many: "Run that lap, run that lap, run, run, run!" Or something like that.

Once the cheering stops, usually midway through the first or second workout, how your exercise program directly affects the life of your spouse or support staff has a significant impact. If you choose to work out in the morning and your spouse is accustomed to your making breakfast for the family in the morning, your exercise program is doomed to failure unless your spouse happens to develop a fondness for pancake flipping. In other words, you and your support staff need to be on the same page as far as schedules, goals, and, most important, priorities. Have frank discussions about why you want to exercise, as well as your goals, fears, and plans, early and often with the support staff. This will help everyone to move in the same direction and will reduce the chances that your support staff will actually sabotage your newfound love of speed walking, or whatever makes you feel better and get more fit. The true support staff will share most of your priorities and will be there to help develop plans to meet both of your needs.

Schedule Time for Exercise

When you start listing all the things you need to accomplish, you probably feel like you're already overloaded and wonder how you're going to fit in exercise. Let's look at a time allotment for a typical week. There are 168 hours in one week. During that week you might, for example,

- sleep 42 to 56 hours,
- commute to work and home 7 to 14 hours,
- work 40 to 60 hours,
- go to church 1 to 3 hours, and
- eat 7 to 14 hours.

That leaves 24 to 72 hours in the week to try to fit in at least 1 hour of exercise. Fitting in the exercise really requires a high level of commitment and some deliberate planning. If you just don't have a large chunk of time in your day to devote to exercise, there are ways to get around that and still fit in your workout.

Here are just a few tips to consider when trying to add more exercise and activity into your day:

- Remember that postexercise hypotension (discussed in chapter 2) can be achieved from exercise bouts as short as 3 minutes, so if you don't have 30 consecutive minutes, exercise for shorter periods multiple times but make sure the total reaches at least 30 minutes.
- Wake up 40 minutes earlier: 5 minutes to get dressed, 30 minutes to exercise, 5 extra minutes.
- Multitask—add a short walk while waiting for soccer practice or music lessons to end.
- Do more yard or house work—it can add up.
- Park in the spot farthest away from the door of the store or your office and walk.

Eliminate Barriers

Start thinking about the reasons you've used to talk yourself out of exercising. These are the barriers that stop you. Write down that part about being too tired and not having enough time. Or the fact that you don't have any safe place to exercise. You might even include the deep fears that you have had for several years about sweating in public or being seen in exercise clothes. You get the idea; we want to identify all the possible barriers in your way first, then we will knock 'em down!

Now let's really think of some creative ways to overcome the barriers and fears in your way. Where can you exercise safely? The mall, at work, around the police station? Remember that the more the merrier—consider exercising with a partner: research shows that when people exercise together, the perceived level of exertion is actually less than the actual level of exertion experienced when you exercise alone. If the clothes issue has you down, pick places or times when few people will see you. You would be surprised how many people begin their workouts at five in the morning for this reason. As we discussed earlier, if time is an issue, consider how you can combine exercise with other activities, like working out with your spouse or kids, or reading, watching TV, or doing other fun things while walking on the treadmill or riding the stationary bike. Remember, this is the creative part of the plan.

Finally, the very last thing to write down is the day and time you plan to begin. Pick the most convenient time in the week for you: Saturday morning at 9:00, or Sunday afternoon at 4:00, or Monday evening at 6:30. Whatever works. Pick the date and time, write it down, and show someone your plan. The power of the written word and peer support will get you going and help keep you going.

It's also important to do your best to plan for and avoid the inevitable roadblocks that will stand in the way of your exercise success. For example, what will you do if it starts raining about 10 minutes before your 20-mile bike ride? Or if you have an unexpected meeting that overlaps your regular morning walk? Or if you get to the pool for your long swim workout and find that the pool has been closed for public health reasons? What are you going to do? What is the backup fitness plan for the day? Are you going to put on the rain gear and go for a ride anyway, or just go for a fast walk or jog in the rain instead? Is there an indoor track nearby, or a mall where you can do a dry fast walk? Perhaps, because you love cycling so much, you purchased a low-cost trainer to throw your bike onto to do the ride in your living room in front of the TV. However you decide to adjust, have your plan in writing beforehand and you will be more likely to get your workout in on the day of an unexpected roadblock.

Mix It Up

Boredom is another motivation stopper. Sticking to the same type of exercise time after time can get dull for some people. But the beauty of committing to an active lifestyle is that there are a variety of activities you can enjoy to reap the benefits of a lower blood pressure. Your very simple goal will be to progress your level of activity so that a workout of any type—badminton, walking, square dancing, golf, swimming, mowing the lawn, Pilates—adds up to a daily caloric expenditure of about 300 calories. That's about 2,000 calories extra per week! Keep it up and your old friends will not recognize you at your next reunion because you are so trim. (See chapter 4 for more on how to measure the intensity of these different activities.)

Avoid Injury

Nothing puts the brakes on a well-planned, properly motivated exercise program like an exercise-induced overuse injury. An injury certainly will put a screeching halt to any well-planned fitness program, which is just one reason why you should pay attention to injury prevention. There has been a saying among NFL football players for years that everyone plays hurt, but few play with injuries. What's the difference? "Hurt" is usually due to relative overuse. The most common example is temporary muscle soreness. If you've exercised, or even if you've temporarily stepped up your weekend activity—raking leaves all day Saturday, for example—chances are you've experienced the delayed-onset muscle soreness (DOMS) we talked about in chapter 5. DOMS is temporary and occurs as a result of using muscles in a way the muscles are not accustomed to. It usually begins within 48 hours of the activity and lasts for four or five days afterward. The best news is that the pain improves with activity, so a good rule of thumb when judging whether you are hurt or truly injured is to try some activity for at least 10 to 15 minutes—that is, if you can do anything! If you can do it and the pain and stiffness improve, stay with it—it's DOMS. If it becomes worse, count yourself as another statistic and contact your doctor or a sports medicine physician for an evaluation of the problem.

Remember that the best way to reduce your risk of overuse injury is to not increase your training volume by more than 10 percent per week. Overuse injuries typically are those nagging tendinitis issues, muscle injuries, or even stress fractures that result from doing too much too soon. Different from the more common delayed-onset muscle soreness, which comes from adding more activity than you are used to doing, overuse injuries generally are more serious and probably end more exercise programs than anything else. The training programs in this book are designed to increase training volume at a rate of 10 percent or less. Table 8.1 shows how much a certain percentage of increase in intensity raises your chance of injury.

Table 8.1   Chance of Injury Based on Training Volume Increase

Percentage of increase per week	Intensity	Workout duration (minutes)	Weekly calories	Injury in
10–15	1 MET	2–3	40–50	6–8 weeks
50	2.5 METs	10–15	200	2–3 weeks
100	5 METs	20–30	400	1 week
>100	>5 METs	>30	>400	Days

Based on a 70-kilogram beginner with a functional capacity of 10 METs using a 20- to 30-minute initial plan.

Adapted from "Overuse Injuries," by WA Scott, in *ACSM's Essentials of Sports Medicine,* edited by RE Sallis and F. Massimino, 1997, with permission of Elsevier.

What to do in the short term? For pain that continues beyond the temporary soreness, overuse injuries are managed in the same manner as an acute injury, such as an ankle or knee sprain—use the RICE method, detailed in the following sidebar.

RICE: Rest, Ice, Compression, and Elevation

The first thing to do is **rest**. If, for some reason, this is not possible, then at least get *relative rest*—that is, reduce the amount, intensity, and frequency of your exercise program until the injury is under control.

Ice is good for everything that ails you—except frostbite. In order to reduce pain and swelling, regardless of how long it has been since the onset of pain, apply ice and not heat. Ice will always serve as a localized anesthetic by constricting local blood vessels and temporarily numbing the local sensory nerves that seem hell-bent on making your life miserable. Heat, although it may help an area feel better initially, opens localized blood vessels and can contribute to the amount of localized swelling, thus making the pain and stiffness associated with most injuries worse.

Compression, like ice, helps to reduce the effects of localized swelling by squeezing out excess inflammatory fluid away from the injured areas. Various elastic wraps, braces, or bandages can provide compression. Be careful not to apply it too tightly, or else the injured area at best does not get better or at worst turns gangrenous. Always wrap from the bottom up—or start the farthest away from the heart and wrap toward the injured area and toward the heart. This will prevent that squeezed-out fluid from the injured site from pooling downstream and creating more problems. Pneumatic pressure devices are an excellent form of injury therapy because they massage, or gradually compress, the fluid out of the injured area back into the body's circulation. Some of these devices even provide ice at the same time to an injured area.

Once that sore leg is resting on ice and wrapped, **elevate** it. Prop it up, not just on the couch or a footstool, but above the heart, again to promote more circulation of localized inflammatory fluids to other areas of the body that are more readily available to handle a difficult load. Unless the limb or injured area is elevated, improvement from injury is slow.

Logging Your Progress

"Talk is cheap. Always get it in writing."

This is good advice for many important deals in life. Why should the deal you make for your health, with yourself—or someone else—be any less significant? The value of seeing what your goals and expectations are with regard to your new fitness program cannot be overestimated. A daily visual reminder of how and why you are exercising is a popular form of motivation for many a fitness buff. Many will write a "contract," either with themselves or someone else. In exchange for your regular exercise adherence, you agree to buy yourself a new portable MP3 player or something like that. If you can find someone else to agree to buy it for you in exchange for your regular exercise participation, more power to you. Either way, put it in writing.

In addition to writing down your goals, it is also important to follow your regular progress by recording a few highlights of each workout. Suggestions on exercise diaries range from the old-fashioned notepad and pencil to fancy computer programs that prompt you on what information to record and store. If you're a creative computer programmer and want to make your own, any database or spreadsheet program will work. A sample log would look something like that shown in figure 8.1.

Use your exercise log to plan and track your progress. If you are a planner, schedule which activity you plan to do on a given day and decide how long the activity needs to be to burn 300 big ones. By doing this you will not only *feel* more in control of your health, you *will* be in control. You will be able to recognize potential under- or over-exercise periods, which will in turn help you maximize the efficiency of your training schedule. On the other hand, if you are not a planner or note writer by nature, try to record your efforts after the fact. Again, this will help you to remain in control.

Dates: from _____ to _____

Blood pressure: _____

Weight: _____ BMI: _____

Medications/dosage: _____

Goals: _____

_____

_____

Date/ time	Type of exercise	Duration	Distance or weight lifted	Intensity	Target HR	Calories burned	Comments

Figure 8.1 This sample exercise log is set up for recording two or three weeks' exercise on the same log. Then blood pressure, weight, BMI, and goals would be reassessed and a new log made for the next two or three weeks. This can be varied according to your preference.

From *Action Plan for High Blood Pressure* by Jon G. Divine, 2006, Champaign, IL: Human Kinetics.

Maximizing Blood Pressure Benefits

Let's not forget that one of the main goals of your exercise program is to lower your blood pressure. Although it would be nice to lower your pressure to the ideal range within a few workouts, this is not a realistic possibility. You and your doctor should discuss realistic goals for both your blood pressure and body weight, as these will both be affected by perhaps the most influential factor in obtaining fitness goals: how much and how regularly you exercise. I like to suggest to my patients that they keep track of only the amount and frequency of their exercise, because this is something they can directly control. When they come in for check-ups I like to document and record where they are in their workout plan and how well they have stuck to it. It is important to keep in mind that as the miles pass under foot, so too will the fat pounds and millimeters of resting blood pressure.

Monitoring Blood Pressure

Some may prefer to add a section to their exercise diary for monitoring blood pressure. Monitoring blood pressure daily is good for some and not others. Daily variations in blood pressure occur, which means that anyone monitoring pressure might well have a high blood pressure reading one day. This reading could make the person unnecessarily anxious and could even have a direct effect on increasing pressure. If you find this information helpful and not stressful, then daily monitoring is OK for you. Regardless of your anxiety level and temperament, it is best to discuss with your doctor how often to measure your pressure and develop a proactive plan about what to do if the pressure is either too high or too low.

There are several commercially available devices to monitor blood pressure. Again, you should discuss this with your doctor, but most will advise purchasing one and learning how to properly use it. Most are accurate—I often recommend that my patients bring their newly purchased machines to my office and compare its readings to readings obtained with my office monitors.

What makes a good home blood pressure monitor? Nothing beats an experienced blood pressure "taker" with a standard sphygmomanometer and a stethoscope. If you have a family member who is experienced in taking accurate blood pressure readings, this is perhaps the best means of measuring blood pressure. Experienced pros can even check their own pressure accurately with this method. If your loved one is unwilling, or you prefer a more objective, impartial means, then an automatic home device is an alternative. Ideally the machine should be lightweight, durable, and have a results display that is easy to read. Some will also provide heart rate, but this is not an essential feature. The cuff size is important: if you have a large arm, you want to purchase an appropriately sized arm band to use with your new device. Likewise, if you have a smaller arm, a smaller cuff is for you. Some machines will allow you to store your information, which is a worthwhile time-saving feature, with little additional cost. Most monitors are battery operated. *Consumer Reports,* a good resource for product reliability and value, rated several blood pressure monitoring devices in their June 2003 issue.

Measuring blood pressure during exercise is very difficult, even for those with experience. There are no commercially available home blood pressure measuring devices capable of measuring blood pressure automatically during exercise. The best means of measuring exercising blood pressure is to measure it shortly after stopping exercise while not moving. Remember, systolic pressure will be higher during exercise, whereas diastolic pressure should ideally be the same as or lower than resting pressure.

What to Do If Blood Pressure Is Too High

Every patient wants to know how high is too high. The short answer is that any pressure that exceeds 200/110 is a medical emergency and should be evaluated and controlled immediately. Anything less than that is not going to result in dire health consequences, but it can affect your exercise routine. Remember, the systolic pressure elevates with exercise, and the diastolic can also rise. A higher resting pressure reduces the protective "buffer zone" where the pressure can remain without causing harm. As long as your resting pressure is below 140/90, you have a free pass to do whatever you can do. If your pressure is continually above 140/90 despite your positive lifestyle and medication changes, talk to your doctor about how to try to keep the pressure below 140/90. Until your pressure is stabilized you should avoid any type of isometric exercises and reduce the intensity of any aerobic or strength-training exercise.

If you have known end-organ illness—heart disease, kidney disease, retinal disease, or a previous stroke—then your exercise intensity should also be on the low side. Your sustained aerobic exercise intensity should be about 50 to 60 percent of maximum heart rate when you are beginning a new program and no higher than 70 percent of maximum as you gain experience. Weight training should be done with very light weights. Remember to practice proper form, and above all, don't strain to lift anything or hold your breath.

If you are in the minority of persons who are "maxed out" on numerous blood pressure medications and still have problems keeping your pressure down, don't give up. Your doctor may advise you to continue exercising at a low relative intensity such as about 45 to 50 percent of maximum heart rate. This may equate to a brisk walk. The trick for this is to do it daily. It is absolutely essential for you to maintain a daily routine of low-intensity exercise. Evidence has shown that when people with extremely high pressures miss a day of exercise, their pressures can rebound to higher levels. So if you're in the difficult-to-control, high-pressure group, strive for perfect attendance!

Monitoring Heart Rate

The heart rate is your body's speedometer during exercise and strenuous activity. Heart rate during activity is perhaps the most accurate means of measuring the relative intensity of the activity—relative, because what may be an easy 7 MPH jogging pace for an experienced runner is an extremely high-intensity activity for the average, step-off-the-couch newbie exerciser. Keep in mind that to achieve, improve, and maintain fitness your heart rate needs to elevate to and remain at a certain rate for at least 20 to 60 minutes for optimal benefits. Remember from your assessment information that your target exercising heart rate should be between 50 and 85 percent of your actual or predicted maximum heart rate. Too high and you're doing too much, too low and you're not doing enough—it's that simple.

Feeling your exercising pulse is the least expensive means of monitoring your heart rate and is easier than most people imagine. First, locate the pulse in your neck (carotid artery area) or at your wrist (see figures 8.2*a* and *b*). Then begin to count your pulse for 15 seconds (use a stopwatch). You may need to slow down your exercise while doing this, but you don't need to stop. Most exercise heart rates are reported as beats per minute, so multiply your 15-second count by 4, and there you have it: your exercising heart rate in beats per minute (BPM). With experience, you will learn what your target heart rate for 15 seconds is without doing the mental

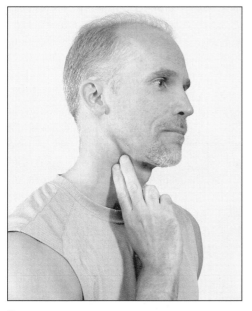
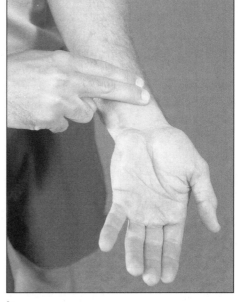

a   b

Figure 8.2   Taking pulse *(a)* at the neck and *(b)* at the wrist.

arithmetic of converting to BPM. Of course, you will also need to know what your 15-second target heart rate range should be as well.

Heart rate monitors range in price from $20 to over $300. You get what you pay for as far as accuracy and features. The site for pulse taking varies by device: some take at the fingertip, others at the ear lobe, others at the wrist. Devices that are more expensive rely on a telemetric measuring and transmitting device, such as a chest strap used with a wristwatch that acts as a receiving and storage device. This frees you up from slowing down and finding your pulse to count. Some are equipped with alarms that alert you when you either exceed your heart rate or need to pick up the pace. All report heart rate in BPM, so no need for the calculating and remembering. The more expensive monitors also have a downloadable feature that is very handy for logging workout intensities.

Spurring Improvement

Well, here we are near the end of the book. Perhaps by now you have gotten into your program for six months or so, and you feel that you would like to take this up a notch and improve. Well, let me be the first to say, good job! Statistically, you have beaten the fitness dropout odds by making it to six months of exercising at least three times a week. Over 50 percent of people beginning a workout program will have dropped out over the same amount of time. At this point, you are in the minority of those who have committed the amount of time and energy required to make a difference in your health. By taking charge of your blood pressure reduction program, you more than likely have reduced your resting systolic blood pressure by over 20 mmHg. By the way, now might be a good time to see your doctor again, because that medicine you're taking to keep your pressure low may need to be adjusted to reflect your newfound form of self-mastery!

To improve your performance in your chosen sport you will need to vary the exercise intensity. In order to increase the demands on your system you will need to gradually add enough overload to allow your body to progressively adapt and thus perform better. Runners who want to run faster need to run faster on training runs. Swimmers need to add fast swimming intervals to a regular steady pace used for training to improve endurance. The programs listed in chapters 4 and 5 have enough flexibility to allow many novices to begin an exercise program. After six months or so, many may choose to stay at the same level. If you want to increase and perhaps improve your fitness level, experiment with increasing intensity per workout simply by walking, running, swimming, or cycling 3 to 5 percent faster. Another option is to add one more workout per week. Adding the workout is even better if you add a different activity. Begin by doing the additional workout for only half the time of your usual workout and gradually increase by about 5 minutes per workout

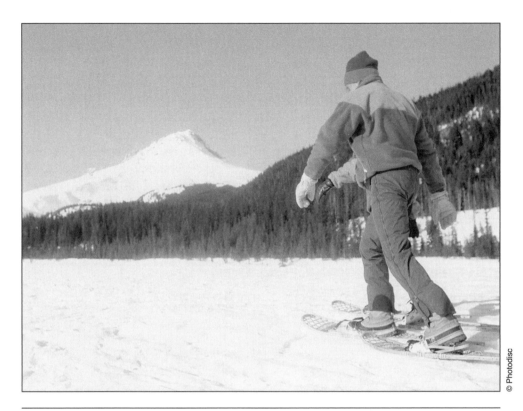

© Photodisc

Adding diverse exercise activities into your routine—showshoeing, for example—keeps you interested and helps prevent injury.

per week until you reach the same duration as the other workouts in the week. Diversity in your routine is another way to prevent injury. Remember, the most important rule about preventing injury is to not increase your mileage, pace, exercise time, or number of workouts by more than 10 percent per week.

Perhaps the best way to improve any skill is to establish a relationship with a qualified coach. A good coach will be able to assess your current level of ability and work with you on improving. There are several ways to locate coaches in your area. Ask people you work out with. Check at a local college—many coaches at small colleges have assistants who are more than willing to take out athletes to train. There might be a fee for their time; this should be established upfront so there are no financial surprises acting as roadblocks in the path of your success. The Internet can also be a very good source of coaching information, although individualized programs found there may also require a fee. Finally, there are several other "how-to" books on your sport. After all, if you have met your fitness goals solely from reading and taking the advice in this book, then books are a good source of information for you.

Summary

A diagnosis of high blood pressure doesn't have to be the end to an active life. On the contrary, great potential exists if you take advantage of physical activity and exercise to lower high blood pressure and maintain a healthy pressure. In addition to directly affecting blood pressure, exercise—through its many general health benefits—helps to lower risk for conditions that contribute to high blood pressure, such as obesity and diabetes. Sometimes medication will still be necessary, but many times it can be avoided with healthy lifestyle modifications. I hope through this book you are encouraged to create or modify an exercise program and healthy eating plan to take control of your blood pressure and health!

ACTION PLAN:
MONITORING PROGRESS AND SPURRING IMPROVEMENT

- ☐ Corral your "support staff"—family and friends who know your goals and will support you as you achieve them.
- ☐ Examine your schedule and plan times to exercise, even if it means being creative by adding exercise into already-scheduled events.
- ☐ Make a list of barriers that keep you from exercising, and identify ways to conquer each barrier.
- ☐ Experiment with different forms of exercise to keep yourself interested—just remember to maintain the same amount of energy expenditure per week.
- ☐ Remember to never increase your activity by more than 10 percent over the previous week's exercise.
- ☐ Learn how to deal with injuries and how to know when the soreness is nothing to worry about.
- ☐ Record your goals and develop an exercise log format that works for you.
- ☐ Monitor your blood pressure and heart rate during exercise, and have a plan ready in case your pressure rises too high.

APPENDIX:
BODY MASS INDEX VALUES

Body Mass Index Values

To use the table, find the appropriate height in the left-hand column labeled Height. Move across to your weight. The number at the top of the column is the BMI at that height and weight. Pounds have been rounded off.

BMI	19	20	21	22	23	24	25	26	27	28	29	30
Height (inches)	Body weight (pounds)											
58	91	96	100	105	110	115	119	124	129	134	138	143
59	94	99	104	109	114	119	124	128	133	138	143	148
60	97	102	107	112	118	123	128	133	138	143	148	153
61	100	106	111	116	122	127	132	137	143	148	153	158
62	104	109	115	120	126	131	136	142	147	153	158	164
63	107	113	118	124	130	135	141	146	152	158	163	169
64	110	116	122	128	134	140	145	151	157	163	169	174
65	114	120	126	132	138	144	150	156	162	168	174	180
66	118	124	130	136	142	148	155	161	167	173	179	186
67	121	127	134	140	146	153	159	166	172	178	185	191
68	125	131	138	144	151	158	164	171	177	184	190	197
69	128	135	142	149	155	162	169	176	182	189	196	203
70	132	139	146	153	160	167	174	181	188	195	202	209
71	136	143	150	157	165	172	179	186	193	200	208	215
72	140	147	154	162	169	177	184	191	199	206	213	221
73	144	151	159	166	174	182	189	197	204	212	219	227
74	148	155	163	171	179	186	194	202	210	218	225	233
75	152	160	168	176	184	192	200	208	216	224	232	240
76	156	164	172	180	189	197	205	213	221	230	238	246

BMI	31	32	33	34	35	36	37	38	39	40	41	42
Height (inches)	Body weight (pounds)											
58	148	153	158	162	167	172	177	181	186	191	196	201
59	153	158	163	168	173	178	183	188	193	198	203	208
60	158	163	168	174	179	184	189	194	199	204	209	215
61	164	169	174	180	185	190	195	201	206	211	217	222
62	169	175	180	186	191	196	202	207	213	218	224	229
63	175	180	186	191	197	203	208	214	220	225	231	237
64	180	186	192	197	204	209	215	221	227	232	238	244
65	186	192	198	204	210	216	222	228	234	240	246	252
66	192	198	204	210	216	223	229	235	241	247	253	260
67	198	204	211	217	223	230	236	242	249	255	261	268
68	203	210	216	223	230	236	243	249	256	262	269	276
69	209	216	223	230	236	243	250	257	263	270	277	284
70	216	222	229	236	243	250	257	264	271	278	285	292
71	222	229	236	243	250	257	265	272	279	286	293	301
72	228	235	242	250	258	265	272	279	287	294	302	309
73	235	242	250	257	265	272	280	288	295	302	310	318
74	241	249	256	264	272	280	287	295	303	311	319	326
75	248	256	264	272	279	287	295	303	311	319	327	335
76	254	263	271	279	287	295	304	312	320	328	336	344

BMI	43	44	45	46	47	48	49	50	51	52	53	54
Height (inches)	Body weight (pounds)											
58	205	210	215	220	224	229	234	239	244	248	253	258
59	212	217	222	227	232	237	242	247	252	257	262	267
60	220	225	230	235	240	245	250	255	261	266	271	276
61	227	232	238	243	248	254	259	264	269	275	280	285
62	235	240	246	251	256	262	267	273	278	284	289	295
63	242	248	254	259	265	270	278	282	287	293	299	304
64	250	256	262	267	273	279	285	291	296	302	308	314
65	258	264	270	276	282	288	294	300	306	312	318	324
66	266	272	278	284	291	297	303	309	315	322	328	334
67	274	280	287	293	299	306	312	319	325	331	338	344
68	282	289	295	302	308	315	322	328	335	341	348	354
69	291	297	304	311	318	324	331	338	345	351	358	365
70	299	306	313	320	327	334	341	348	355	362	369	376
71	308	315	322	329	338	343	351	358	365	372	379	386
72	316	324	331	338	346	353	361	368	375	383	390	397
73	325	333	340	348	355	363	371	378	386	393	401	408
74	334	342	350	358	365	373	381	389	396	404	412	420
75	343	351	359	367	375	383	391	399	407	415	423	431
76	353	361	369	377	385	394	402	410	418	426	435	443

Reprinted from the CDC (Centers for Disease Control and Prevention).

BIBLIOGRAPHY

ALLHAT Officers and Coordinators for the ALLHAT Collaborative Research Group. 2002. Major outcomes in high-risk hypertensive patients randomized to angiotensin converting enzyme inhibitor or calcium channel blocker vs diuretic: The Antihypertensive and Lipid-Lowering Treatment to Prevent Heart Attack Trial. *Journal of the American Medical Association* 288:2981-2997.

American College of Sports Medicine. 2004. Position Stand: Exercise and hypertension. *Medicine & Science in Sports & Exercise* 36:533-553.

American College of Sports Medicine. 2002. Position Stand: Progression models in resistance training for healthy adults. *Medicine & Science in Sports & Exercise* 34: 364-380.

American College of Sports Medicine. 2000. *ACSM's guidelines for exercise testing and prescription.* 6th ed. Baltimore: Lippincott Williams & Wilkins.

American College of Sports Medicine. 1998. Position Stand: The recommended quantity and quality of exercise for developing and maintaining cardiorespiratory and muscular fitness, and flexibility in healthy adults. *Medicine & Science in Sports & Exercise* 30:975-991.

American College of Sports Medicine. 1998. Position Stand: Exercise and physical activity for older adults. *Medicine & Science in Sports & Exercise* 30:992-1008.

American College of Sports Medicine. 1997. *ACSM's exercise management for persons with chronic diseases and disabilities.* Champaign, IL: Human Kinetics.

American College of Sports Medicine. 1995. *ACSM's guidelines for exercise testing and prescription.* 5th ed. Baltimore: Lippincott Williams & Wilkins.

American Heart Association. 2005. High blood pressure statistics. [Online]. Available: www.americanheart.org/presenter.jhtml?identifier=212 [June 6, 2005].

Appel, L.J., T.J. Moore, E. Obarzanek, W.M. Vollmer, L.P. Svetkey, F.M. Sacks, G.A. Bray, T.M. Vogt, J.A. Cutler, M.M. Windhauser, P.H. Lin, and N. Karanja. 1997. A clinical trial of the effects of dietary patterns on blood pressure. DASH Collaborative Research Group. *New England Journal of Medicine* 336:1117-1124.

Borg, G.A. 1982. Psychological basis of physical education. *Medicine & Science in Sports & Exercise* 14:377.

Braith, R.W., J.E. Graves, S.H. Leggett, and M.L. Pollock. 1993. Effect of training on the relationship between maximal and submaximal strength. *Medicine & Science in Sports & Exercise* 25:132.

Burke, E.R. 2002. *Serious cycling.* 2nd ed. Champaign, IL: Human Kinetics.

Chobanian, A.V., G.L. Bakris, H.R. Black, W.C. Cushman, L.A. Green, J.L. Izzo, D.W. Jones, B.J. Materson, S. Oparil, J.T. Wright, E.J. Roccella; Joint National Committee on Prevention, Detection, Evaluation, and Treatment of High Blood Pressure. National Heart, Lung, and Blood Institute; National High Blood Pressure Education Program Coordinating Committee. 2003. The seventh report of the Joint National Committee on Prevention, Detection, Evaluation, and Treatment of High Blood Pressure: the JNC 7 report. *Journal of the American Medical Association* 289:2560-2572.

Chobanian, A.V., and M. Hill. 2000. National Heart, Lung, and Blood Institute Workshop on Sodium and Blood Pressure: A critical review of current scientific evidence. *Hypertension* 35:858-863.

Chorley, J.N., J.C. Cianca, J.G. Divine, and T.D. Hew. 2003. Baseline injury risk factors for runners starting a marathon training program. *Clinical Journal of Sports Medicine* 12(1):18-23.

Consumer Reports. 2004. *Buying guide 2004.* Yonkers, NY: Consumers Union.

Fredericson, M., M. Guillet, and L. DeBenedictis. 2000. Quick solutions for iliotibial band syndrome. *Physician and Sports Medicine.* 28 (2).

Gordon, N.F., C.B. Scott, and B.D. Levine. 1997. Comparison of single versus multiple lifestyle interventions: Are the antihypertensive effects of exercise training and diet-induced weight loss additive? *American Journal of Cardiology* 79(6):763-767.

He, J., P.K. Whelton, L.J. Appel, J. Charleston, and M.J. Klag. 2000. Long-term effects of weight loss and dietary sodium reduction on incidence of hypertension. *Hypertension* 35:544-549.

Hines, E. 1999. *Fitness swimming.* Champaign, IL: Human Kinetics.

Johnson, B.L., and J.K. Nelson. 1986. *Practical measurements for evaluation in physical education.* 4th ed. New York: Macmillan.

Joint National Committee on Detection, Evaluation, and Treatment of High Blood Pressure. 1997. The sixth report of the Joint National Committee on prevention, detection, evaluation, and treatment of high blood pressure (JNC VI). *Archives of Internal Medicine* 157(21):2413-2446.

Jones, D.W., L.J. Appel, S.G. Sheps, E.J. Roccella, and C. Lenfant. 2003. Measuring blood pressure accurately: New and persistent challenges. *Journal of the American Medical Association* 289:1027-1030.

Kaplan, N.M., R.B. Deveraux, and H.S. Miller. 1994. Systemic hypertension. ACSM and ACC 26th Bethesda Conference. *Medicine & Science in Sports & Exercise* 26:10, S268-S270.

Kelley, G.A. 1999. Aerobic exercise and resting blood pressure among women: A meta-analysis. *Preventive Medicine* 28:264-275.

Kelley, G.A., and K.S. Kelley. 2000. Progressive resistance exercise and resting blood pressure: A meta-analysis of randomized controlled trials. *Hypertension* 35:838-843.

Kohl, H.W., M.Z. Nichaman, R.F. Frankowski, and S.N. Blair. 1996. Maximal exercise hemodynamics and risk of mortality in apparently healthy men and women. *Medicine & Science in Sports & Exercise* 28:601-609.

Kraul, J., J. Chrastek, and J. Adamirova. 1966. The hypotensive effect of physical activity. In *Prevention of ischemic heart disease: Principles and practice,* ed. W. Rabb, 359-371. Springfield, IL: Charles C. Thomas.

Lee, E.N. 2004. The effects of tai chi exercise program on blood pressure, total cholesterol and cortisol level in patients with essential hypertension. *Taehan Kanho Hakhoe Chi* 34(5):829-837.

MacDonald, L. 1989. Swimming: Fitness afloat—swimming as exercise. *Diabetes Forecast.*

Naughton, J., and R. Haider. 1973. Methods of exercise training. In *Exercise testing and exercise training in coronary heart disease,* ed. J.P. Naughton, H.K. Hellerstein, and I.C. Mohler. New York: Academic Press.

Niedfeldt, M.W. 2002. Managing hypertension in athletes and physically active patients. *American Family Physician* 66:445-452.

Paffenbarger, R.S., R.T. Hyde, A.L. Wing, and C.C. Hsieh. 1986. Physical activity, all-cause mortality, and longevity of college alumni. *New England Journal of Medicine* 314(10): 605-613.

Pescatello, L.S., A.E. Fargo, C.N. Leach, and H.H. Scherzer. 1991. Short-term effect of dynamic exercise on arterial blood pressure. *Circulation* 83(5):1557-1561.

Pollock, M.L., J.H. Wilmore, and S.M. Fox. 1984. *Exercise in health and disease: Evaluation and prescription for prevention and rehabilitation.* Philadelphia: W.B. Saunders.

President's Council on Physical Fitness and Sports. 2003. Physical activity and the Stages of Motivational Readiness for Change model. *Research Digest* Series 4(1):1-8.

Ronda, M.U., A.M. Alves, and F.W. Braga. 2002. Postexercise blood pressure reduction in elderly hypertensive patients. *Journal of the American College of Cardiology* 39: 676-682.

Sacks, F.M., L.P. Svetkey, W.M. Vollmer, L.J. Appel, G.A. Bray, D. Harsha, E. Obarzanek, P.R. Conlin, E.R. Miller, D.G. Simons-Morton, N. Karanja, and P.H. Lin. 2001. Effects on blood pressure of reduced dietary sodium and the Dietary Approaches to Stop Hypertension (DASH) diet. DASH-Sodium Collaborative Research Group. *New England Journal of Medicine* 344:3-10.

Steffen, P.R., A. Sherwood, E. Gullette, A. Georgiades, A. Hinderliter, and J.A. Blumenthal. 2001. Effects of exercise and weight loss on blood pressure during daily life. *Medicine & Science in Sports & Exercise* 33:1635-1640.

Stevens, V.J., E. Obarzanek, N.R. Cook, I.M. Lee, L.J. Appel, D. Smith West, N.C. Milas, M. Mattfeldt-Beman, L. Belden, C. Bragg, M. Millstone, J. Raczynski, A. Brewer, B. Singh, and J. Cohen. 2001. Long-term weight loss and changes in blood pressure: Results of the Trials of Hypertension Prevention, phase II. *Annals of Internal Medicine* 134:1-11.

Sundar, S., S.K. Agrawal, V.P. Singh, S.K. Bhattacharya, K.N. Udupa, and S.K. Vaish. 1984. Role of yoga in management of essential hypertension. *Acta Cardiologica* 39(3):203-208.

Tanji, J.L. 1992. Exercise and the hypertensive athlete. *Clinics in Sports Medicine* 11(2): 291-302.

Trials of Hypertension Prevention Collaborative Research Group. 1997. Effects of weight loss and sodium reduction intervention on blood pressure and hypertension incidence in overweight people with high-normal blood pressure. The Trials of Hypertension Prevention, phase II. *Archives of Internal Medicine* 157:657-667.

Tsai, J.C., W.H. Wang, P. Chan, L.J. Lin, C.H. Wang, B. Tomlinson, M.H. Hsieh, H.Y. Yang, and J.C. Liu. 2003. The beneficial effects of Tai Chi Chuan on blood pressure and lipid profile and anxiety status in a randomized controlled trial. *The Journal of Alternative and Complementary Medicine* 9(5):747-754.

Vijayalakshmi, P., Madanmohan, A.B. Bhavanani, A. Patil, and K. Babu. 2004. Modulation of stress induced by isometric handgrip test in hypertensive patients following yogic relaxation training. *Indian Journal of Physiology and Pharmacology* 48(1):59-64.

Vollmer, W.M., F.M. Sacks, J. Ard, L.J. Appel, G.A. Bray, D.G. Simons-Morton, P.R. Conlin, L.P. Svetkey, T.P. Erlinger, T.J. Moore, and N. Karanja. 2001. Effects of diet and sodium intake on blood pressure: Subgroup analysis of the DASH-sodium trial. DASH-Sodium Trial Collaborative Research Group. *Annals of Internal Medicine* 135:1019-1028.

Wallace, J.P. 2003. Exercise in hypertension: A clinical review. *Sports Medicine* 33:585-598.

Whelton, S.P., A. Chin, X. Xin, and J. He. 2002. Effect of aerobic exercise on blood pressure: A meta-analysis of randomized, controlled trials. *Annals of Internal Medicine* 136(7): 493-503.

Whelton, S.P., J. He, L.J. Appel, J.A. Cutler, S. Havas, T.A. Kotchen, E.J. Roccella, R. Stout, C. Vallbona, M.C. Winston, and J. Karimbakes. 2002. Primary prevention of hypertension: Clinical and public health advisory from the National High Blood Pressure Education Program. *Journal of the American Medical Association* 288:1882-1888.

Xin, X., J. He, M.G. Frontini, L.G. Ogden, O.I. Motsamai, and P.K. Whelton. 2001. Effects of alcohol reduction on blood pressure: A meta-analysis of randomized controlled trials. *Hypertension* 38:1112-1117.

INDEX

Note: The italicized *f* and *t* following page numbers refer to figures and tables, respectively.

ABOUT THE AUTHOR

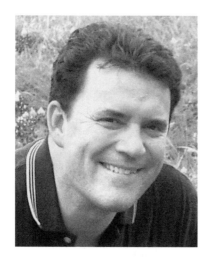

Jon G. Divine, MD, MS, FACSM, is currently associate professor in the department of pediatrics at the University of Cincinnati Medical Center and medical director of the Sports Medicine Biodynamics Center at the Cincinnati Children's Hospital Medical Center. An educator in the sports science field for more than 15 years, Divine also has earned a certificate of added qualifications (CAQ) in sports medicine and a board certification in family medicine. In addition to writing articles for peer-reviewed journals such as *Medicine & Science in Sports & Exercise* and the *Clinical Journal of Sports Medicine,* Divine has lent his expertise to several sports medicine books. He has been certified as an ACSM Exercise Specialist since 1988, served as president of the Texas Chapter of ACSM, and was honored as an ACSM fellow in 2003. Divine also maintains memberships in the American Medical Society for Sports Medicine, American Academy of Family Physicians, and American Medical Association.

Divine resides in Union, Kentucky, with his wife, Leigh Ann, and their two children.

ABOUT ACSM

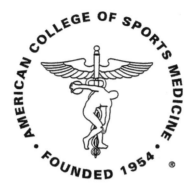

The **American College of Sports Medicine (ACSM)** is more than the world's leader in the scientific and medical aspects of sports and exercise; it is an association of people and professions exploring the use of medicine and exercise to make life healthier for all people.

Since 1954, ACSM has been committed to the promotion of physical activity and the diagnosis, treatment, and prevention of sport-related injuries. With more than 20,000 international, national, and regional chapter members in 80 countries, ACSM is internationally known as the leading source of state-of-the-art research and information on sports medicine and exercise science. Through ACSM, health and fitness professionals representing a variety of disciplines work to improve the quality of life for people around the world through health and fitness research, education, and advocacy.

A large part of ACSM's mission is devoted to public awareness and education about the positive aspects of physical activity for people of all ages and from all walks of life. ACSM's physicians, researchers, and educators have created tools for the public, ranging in scope from starting an exercise program to avoiding or treating sport injuries.

ACSM's National Center is located in Indianapolis, Indiana, widely recognized as the amateur sports capital of the nation. To learn more about ACSM, visit www.acsm.org.

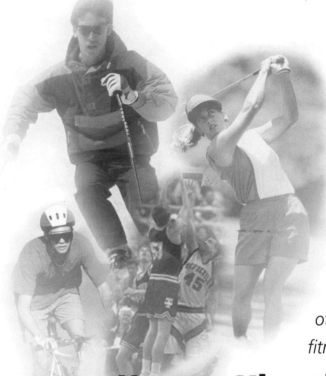

*You'll find
other outstanding
fitness resources at*

www.HumanKinetics.com

In the U.S. call

1-800-747-4457

Australia.............................	08 8277 1555
Canada	1-800-465-7301
Europe......................	+44 (0) 113 255 5665
New Zealand..................	0064 9 448 1207

HUMAN KINETICS
The Premier Publisher for Sports & Fitness
P.O. Box 5076 • Champaign, IL 61825-5076 USA